Research: Some Ground Rules

J. S. P. LUMLEY
Professor of Vascular Surgery
Vascular Unit
St. Bartholomew's Hospital
London

and

WALTER BENJAMIN
Consultant Statistician

OXFORD NEW YORK TOKYO
OXFORD UNIVERSITY PRESS
1994

Oxford University Press, Walton Street, Oxford OX2 6DP

Oxford   New York
Athens   Auckland   Bangkok   Bombay
Calcutta   Cape Town   Dar es Salaam   Delhi
Florence   Hong Kong   Istanbul   Karachi
Kuala Lumpur   Madras   Madrid   Melbourne
Mexico City   Nairobi   Paris   Singapore
Taipei   Tokyo   Toronto
and associated companies in
Berlin   Ibadan

Oxford is a trade mark of Oxford University Press

Published in the United States
by Oxford University Press Inc., New York

A catalogue record for this book is available from the British Library

Library of Congress Cataloging in Publication Data available

ISBN 0 19 854823 0 (Hbk)
ISBN 0 19 854822 2 (Pbk)

Typeset by
EXPO Holdings, Malaysia
Printed in Great Britain by
Redwood Books, Trowbridge, Wilts

Preface

Individuals entering the research field are drawn from various disciplines and have to acquire many new skills. Some are fortunate enough to enter departments with well-established research programmes and receive a systematic orientation and introduction. Others, however, waste valuable time and energy following many unrewarding pathways. This text is intended to reduce the frustrations for the novice researcher and also outline what they should ask of supervisors, colleagues, and others in the research field. It presents the concepts and principles of research, and advises on how to set out, implement, and complete a research project in an enjoyable and rewarding fashion. Emphasis is given to the practical aspects of a research project, and flow charts are included to guide and indicate the various stages of a research programme. Consideration is given to what students and supervisors should expect of each other.

The initial chapters consider what research involves, the stages of planning, and the necessary fields of study. Sections on human and animal research consider ethical problems and the appropriateness of experimental subjects. Experimental design and surveys are linked to the chapters on statistical analysis, and a practical biological approach is taken. Statistical analysis causes unnecessary aggravation for the uninitiated. This section considers why statistics are needed, the language of the discipline, the rules for dealing with samples, and how to examine for similarities and differences in surveys and experiments. Flow charts indicate how to choose a statistical test, but emphasis is given to the need to discuss the design and analysis of an experiment or survey with a qualified statistician: this section will help such a discussion. Chapters on the presentation of research material provide advice on delivering papers and posters to learned societies, and writing articles and theses. The preparation of illustrative material for all forms of presentation is considered collectively, emphasizing the different requirements for the various modalities. The final chapters consider other diverse writing requirements of the research worker, including grant applications, interviews, and job applications.

The book is not intended as a substitute for regular discussions with interested experts and senior colleagues: new research workers must always be on the lookout for courses and literature relevant to their activities. Although the book presents only one way of approaching a research appointment, it does highlight common problems and their management, and provides a practical guide for all biomedical research workers.

London
January 1994

J. S. P. L.
W. B.

Contents

Section B: Data collection and analysis   61

Section A:
The essentials of biomedical research

1. Principles and practice of research

Overview

Few words portray such a wide variety of images as the term research. It carries a certain mystique; it is often used to impress and can bring an unchallenged halt to a conversation, as though it were an end point in itself. It may also carry with it a feeling of dread and uncertainty to those about to undertake a research position. However, this is a fear of the unknown and this introductory section is intended to allay these anxieties, clarify misconceptions, and indicate that research has very clearly defined boundaries. Research is no more than the process of asking questions and answering them by survey or experiment in an organized way. Although these principles can be applied by every thinking person, there are well-tried pathways and a knowledge of some basic rules greatly facilitates any beginner in this field. A great deal of research is undertaken on part-time projects outside university departments, possibly without skilled direction. This text is intended for individuals taking this approach as well as those fortunate enough to be setting out on a period of full-time research with appropriate supervision. A period of full-time research is advised to acquire an insight into a range of research techniques. It begins with the choice of institution, field, supervisor, and topic, and a comprehensive period of background reading. Once a question and the hypothesis (suggested answer) have been formulated, the method of investigation, with its appropriate statistical form of analysis, are defined. The proposed method of testing the hypothesis is tried out with a pilot study before carrying out and analysing the definitive project. Once meaningful conclusions have been obtained they should be reported to the appropriate audience.

This book is intended to open up the world of research to the reader. Each stage of the research process is described fully and simply, by setting out the main principles and providing a detailed operational guide; thus providing the apprentice with a high degree of independence, the basis for fruitful discussions with the supervisor, and the likelihood of a successful outcome. Section A takes the researcher through the research process as a whole, so that he or she can understand what it is all about, why it is important, and how the different parts fit together: they can also make up their minds whether it is something they really want to do. If it is, they will have sufficient information to get started and map out their time during the research period, ensuring that it is used to good effect. The flow chart in Fig. 1.1 summarizes these stages. Section A also discusses specific aspects of biomedical research with respect to the use of humans and animals, and necessary safety

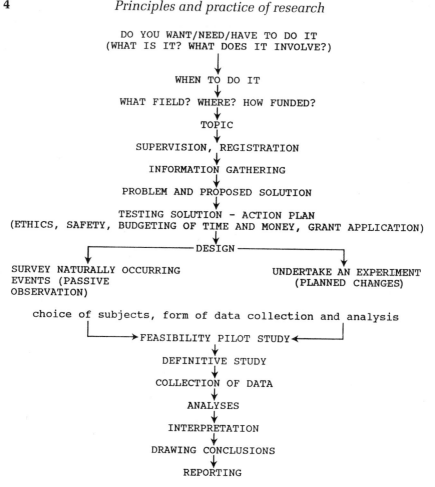

```
          DO YOU WANT/NEED/HAVE TO DO IT
          (WHAT IS IT? WHAT DOES IT INVOLVE?)
                         │
                         ▼
                   WHEN TO DO IT
                         │
             WHAT FIELD? WHERE? HOW FUNDED?
                         │
                       TOPIC
                         │
              SUPERVISION, REGISTRATION
                         │
               INFORMATION GATHERING
                         │
             PROBLEM AND PROPOSED SOLUTION
                         │
               TESTING SOLUTION - ACTION PLAN
     (ETHICS, SAFETY, BUDGETING OF TIME AND MONEY, GRANT APPLICATION)
                         │
        ┌────────────────── DESIGN ──────────────────┐
        ▼                                            ▼
  SURVEY NATURALLY OCCURRING              UNDERTAKE AN EXPERIMENT
  EVENTS (PASSIVE                         (PLANNED CHANGES)
  OBSERVATION)

     choice of subjects, form of data collection and analysis
        └──────▶ FEASIBILITY PILOT STUDY ◀──────┘
                         │
                  DEFINITIVE STUDY
                         │
                 COLLECTION OF DATA
                         │
                      ANALYSES
                         │
                   INTERPRETATION
                         │
                DRAWING CONCLUSIONS
                         │
                     REPORTING
```

Fig. 1.1 Flow chart for the prospective researcher.

measures. This first chapter explains, by using examples, why a structured approach is needed for posing questions and testing hypotheses. The chapter then goes on to explain the advantage of a full-time apprenticeship to learn the necessary skills.

What is research?

The aquisition of knowledge is a continuous process from birth; an individual exploring the environment and asking questions. Information is provided by parents, associates, and teachers and is supplemented by reading books, magazines, newspapers, and other media. As an individual's knowledge increases, questions become more complex and answers come from experts, reference books, and specialized journals. Awareness grows that answers are often unsatisfactory, being incomplete and confused, inaccurate, or nonexistent. Research is the examination of these limits of knowledge; assessing what is known up to that point, defining unanswered questions and devising ways of answering them in an organized and meaningful way. Research is not something which should be confined to university departments; it is within the capability of, and should be undertaken by, every thinking person. Explanations can be suggested and tested out on many of the unanswered questions around us in every day living.

What does it involve?

The first requirement is an enquiring mind, in order to recognize that there are questions needing answers. The next step is to define an unanswered question or questions. This requires careful thinking around the problem. A simple problem (although you will soon realize that this adjective is rarely appropriate) may be that you are not sure what food to provide for a puppy you have just been given. The advice obtained from the pet shop, food shops, friends, posters, and television advertisements has provided conflicting opinions. Although the question is what is the best food product? 'Best' can be interpreted in many ways. The reader is invited to consider five criteria: the cost, availability, dog owners' preference, puppy's preference, and nutritional value. Existing information such as manufacturer's literature and articles in dog magazines may suggest that the product KPH (Keeps Puppies Happy) is the best buy and this hypothesis can be investigated (researched) for the five chosen criteria.

Cost and availability of KPH

The relative cost and availability of KPH can be conveniently assessed together, by means of a *survey*. Surveys document existing events and opinions, often using a questionnaire. The *questionnaire* is designed listing all dog food products manufactured. Cost and availability can vary in different shops and regions and there may be cut price offers and special deals with bulk buying. Cost and availability may also vary at different times of the year. Examples of this type of survey in medical practice are the cost and availability of drugs.

Owners' preference

Owners' preference for KPH also be examined by a survey. Here a more comprehensive questionnaire may be required, as owners are also influenced by the other factors, such as the smell, convenience for serving, and the subsequent ease of cleaning dishes and utensils. Preference may be complicated by KPH being available in different forms. The number of different factors for assessment may become very large and their relative importance to different puppy owners may vary and require some form of grading. Opinions and preference may also be influenced by a recent advertising campaign or an introductory offer. A questionnaire can therefore become very complex and this has to be balanced with the likelihood of it being completed and the benefits which are likely to be obtained from the additional information.

Two further concepts develop from these considerations. The first is the value of a *pilot study*. This is preliminary examination of a questionnaire on a small number of puppy owners to see if it is acceptable, whether it works and if they think it could be improved. Pilot studies form an important part of more complex research projects and often markedly influence their subsequent form. The second consideration is how the large number of pieces of information obtained from complex questionnaires are to be *analysed*. The design and analysis of surveys and experiments is part of the study of *statistics*. This is an exacting and rewarding field that the researcher needs to study. Although the involvement of a statistician is advisable when planning and analysing large investigations, it is important that all researchers understand the logic behind statistical techniques. Equivalent questions about medical products can assess doctors' preferences for drugs or specific treatments in the management of different diseases. When compiling such a list you may be surprised at the similarity of the questions with those in the above paragraph.

Puppies' preference

It is common to be told that 'seven out of 10 dogs prefer a particular food product'. Obtaining similar figures for KPH will provide some insight as to the meaning of such a statement. This could mean that seven out of 10 specifically chosen puppies prefer KPH or it could mean that 70 per cent of *all* puppies prefer KPH. The statement thus depends on the type of study being reported and the discerning owner would be wise to find out how many dogs were tested and how they were chosen. A puppy's preference could be taken as synonymous with owner's preference, but we have already seen that the latter is subject to outside influences, such as cost, availability, introductory offers, and advertising campaigns. When assessing a puppy's preference it should be stated whether this is in relation to all available food products or, for example, those within a set price range, or foods specifically produced for puppies.

If only one puppy is tested the result is only relevant to that particular puppy. Similarly, if only KPH and one other food product are used, the findings are only relevent to these two foods. For the information to be more widely applicable the study must be carried out on more than one puppy and a decision made as to how many food products are to be tested. Note, however, that the larger the number of puppies and the more food products tested, the higher the expense, and the more time needed to complete the investigation. In practice, the researcher studies a sample from the population. The population in this case being all puppies. A sample must be truly representative of the population from which it is drawn. To explain the problems involved, just two food products will be considered. The procedure is to design an experiment so that *factors other than the two foodstuffs do not influence the result*. Possible extraneous factors influencing the results include the age, weight, and breed of puppy, the order and freedom of choice of food product, the number of exposures and how hungry each puppy is at the time of testing. The experiment should exclude or even out the effect of these extraneous factors: the principle is that of *controlling* an experiment. The variables that cannot be evened out or excluded must be *randomized*, to eliminate all extraneous bias. Methods for comparing chosen factors in a controlled way are considered in Chapter 13.

Another important principle to apply whenever possible, is that the assessor should be unaware of which food products are being offered to each puppy (*blind assessment*). A puppy might choose a particular food product by chance alone, but sufficient repeated *unbiased* exposures will help to decide whether any real difference exists or not. However, the criteria for deciding what constitutes a *meaningful difference* must be laid down before the start of an experiment. *Statistical tests* are available to analyse every experimental design. Examples of research into consumer preference are legion. Every food manufacturer has to take into account animal or human preference. In drug therapy this is more under the control of the clinician; but he or she must still take into account patient acceptability and the side effects of a drug or treatment regime.

Nutrition

The criteria for assessing nutrition may be complex; weight gain will be one important consideration. This will vary in different breeds and even in different litter mates, without necessarily indicating a beneficial or detrimental effect. The well-being of an animal may need a skilled judge of breed or a veterinary surgeon for assessment. Other possible factors are energy level, changes of blood chemistry, and resistance to infection. Another consideration that comes into much human and animal research is the *ethics* of an experiment. This could apply if a puppy was not developing satisfactorily—a decision would have to be made whether the experiment should be abandoned. The detailed evaluation of products is an essential requirement for all drug manufacturers, who have to satisfy the legal, as well as the ethical, requirements of each country in which they wish to market their product. The monitoring of therapeutic, as well as other systemic, effects of every new drug is mandatory. These studies should include tests for *compliance* and the pharmacokinetic properties of the product.

Conclusions from KPH study

To say KPH is the best puppy foodstuff, one has to compare it with what else is available. To do this, one undertakes either a survey or an experiment. Surveys examine existing events and opinions. An experiment is designed to test the hypothesis that KPH is best. This is carried out in a controlled way, by excluding, randomizing, or equating extraneous factors. This enables the researcher to compare

KPH with other foodstuffs and demonstrate any differences. As one cannot examine every puppy, investigations are carried out on representative samples drawn from the population. The science of statistics is used in designing and interpreting the results of surveys and experiments. This enables the researcher to estimate how likely sample results represent the population from which they are drawn. In general, the bigger the sample size, the more confident the researcher can be that this generalization is justified. There may be a clear cut result in favour of KPH or another product. Alternatively the extent of any difference may be small and of no consequence.

What to do with the results

Having completed all the work, one has to decide what to do with the information, and how to inform other pet owners, and the manufacturers, shops, and breeder who have been involved. Manufacturers are unlikely to publish bad results of their product, but they should be interested in the results of well-controlled studies and may modify their product accordingly. Points of marked difference should be publicized and there is a moral obligation to publish information on food products which could adversely affect puppies. Letters to newspapers and dog magazines are additional ways of publicizing ones findings, but legal advice should be sought if there is any danger of court action. A large number of general and specialized journals exist which will publish well-controlled studies that provide important information on the positive and negative values of a particular treatment or other regime. However, it is the duty of reviewers and editors to ensure that the research has been undertaken in an organized fashion and that it draws valid conclusions.

Scientific research

The KPH has illustrated some of the problems encountered when attempting to answer questions. A similar enquiring attitude must be applied to one's professional field of interest and should continue throughout one's career. Above all, careful documentation of events allows valuable short- and long-term followup, and analysis of scientific observations. The researcher must have a clear idea of what questions may be asked of the documented information, so that all relevant material is included, and the material and method of information storage are appropriate to subsequent analysis. When groups of workers are involved in a similar field, regular exchange of views and meetings, such as journal clubs allow wider coverage of the literature and valuable times for detailed discussion of articles and the pooling of opinions. In the medical field, studies include detailed examination of unusual individual cases and audit of personal or group activities. These surveys provide critical information on current progress and may direct future clinical practice. Differences noted or suspected may be further examined by experiments set up to assess different management regimes. Clinical and nonclinical research may also be laboratory based, and students should seek out skilled workers who can introduce them to new fields, and direct them in profitable areas of study.

Part-time research should be undertaken by all postgraduates and they should become aware of the joys of investigating problems. Such studies, however, are more enjoyable if they can be brought to completion and become a useful contribution to scientific progress. Surveys on a limited number of subjects can give false information, and it is always dangerous to draw conclusions as to cause and effect. Similarly, experiments must be controlled to obtain meaningful results. Even limited studies must therefore be undertaken in a skilled and organized fashion. This is more likely if early exposure to research is as part of an experienced clinical group, or at least under the direction of an individual trained in research techniques. Fortunately, a large number of clinicians have had training in research techniques and are able to guide the novice in such studies.

Why full-time research?

The reader will have noted the gradual change in emphasis in the last few paragraphs, from an everyday problem to problems studied by the professional, the postgraduate, and other research workers. Although the full-time researcher follows similar pathways, it is important to examine why the trained individual is in a position to carry out a more comprehensive and authoritative study. The benefits of a research training are considered under the four headings of time, training, involvement, and developing a research attitude.

Time

Research takes time and money, and it is desirable (at least in the initial period of research training) that a worker should be free of other heavy work commitments. This freedom allows them to read and think in depth around a topic and go over and over a problem. In this way ideas and theories can be developed. The latter may be in line with current thought or involve more lateral thinking, attacking dogma: novel hypotheses can be formulated even if not compatible with existing knowledge. Time allows the undertaking of meaningful experimentations, testing theories, and alternative explanations.

Training

A training period in research allows an individual to fill any gaps in both research techniques and skills pertinent to the field of study. Information-gathering skills are important to survey literature, and to develop a clear critical approach to all published material (see p. 168). This included papers, monographs, chapters, reviews, and editorials. Well-organized information storage and retrieval systems save a considerable amount of time. The principles of testing theories by surveys and designed experiments must be applied: the trainee must have a clear understanding of the rules for collection and analysis of the data that allow logical and valid conclusions to be made. He or she must be aware of the responsibility to complete and report experiments. The use of pilot studies indicates the feasibility and practicality of a survey or experiment, in terms of obtaining measurable and meaningful results and utilizing the available facilities. The integration of statistics into a research programme is an essential component. The practical and routine application of statistical techniques must be understood, together with its limitations, and the need to take statistical advice at the beginning, rather than at a later stage in a project. The skills of authorship are part and parcel of research: positive and negative results, the limitation of techniques, and the failure to support existing or proposed theories, should be reported in a responsible, coherent, concise, and authoritative way. Other skills which may be required by a biomedical trainee include technical training, an understanding for example of nuclear medicine and genetic engineering, and an introduction to many other branches of pure science.

Involvement

Involvement in full-time research produces an awareness of the need for everyday planning and efficient time utilization. Experience gained in this environment allows insight into the challenge of the unknown, the enthusiasm required in investigation, and the joys and frustrations of this process. A partnership with other research workers provides an awareness of their attitudes and understanding, and exposure to a critical environment. Investigation with workers from different fields provides an appreciation of the multidisciplinary format of present-day research. Team involvement also provides a forum for discussion, challenging concepts and defending theories. Such discussion provides an understanding of the boundaries of knowledge and how these frontiers can be modified.

Development of a research attitude

A period of research training develops in many individuals an insatiable curiosity and a continuous endeavour to provide answers. Success in a field produces a sense of achievement which often culminates in a research career. Above all research teaches an individual the power of self-discipline in undertaking independent work under their own motivation and at their own rate; sustaining impetus and laying down goals to be achieved in specified times. The trained researcher is receptive to change, capable of challenging unfounded claims, providing confident objective opinions and judgements, supported by clear detailed examination and interpretation of the findings.

Who researches?

The desire for answers and the motivation to search for them is not unique to research workers. Previous paragraphs have emphasized that an enquiring mind can be applied to common events and it is an essential requirement for all undergraduate education. Each undergraduate student should be expected to look in detail into an unsolved question, and to develop a thirst for self-education and a critical scientific attitude. Time and money is limited and a topic must be chosen to ensure completion within a set period. As already emphasized, the exploration of uncharted territory requires time, money, and training, and this detailed form of investigation is only available to a privileged few. The choice is usually from those who have proved their ability to collect, assess, and present information at an undergraduate or postgraduate level, and who will therefore make most use of this opportunity. Candidates with good degrees may be offered this option and may look on it as a step to a future career in a university or industrial research environment. A period of research and the acquisition of a postgraduate degree is a mandatory requirement for promotion in many medical disciplines. Progress in a university environment is usually dependent on the publication of research work and linked with its quality.

Summary

1. Re-examine the flow chart in Fig. 1.1 (p. 4).

2. Research has been defined as the process of finding explanations to unanswered questions. This is something every thinking person does, and is not restricted to people labelled as researchers.

3. As shown with the puppy food product KPH, a problem is rarely simple. The key to finding an acceptable answer is in using a structured and disciplined approach which allows proposed hypotheses to be fully assessed. A period of full-time research provides a useful apprenticeship in gaining the skills required.

4. For some individuals the initial period of research is so fulfilling, they continue it as a career. For others, the experience gained enables them to question research colleagues critically and confidently, and not to be trapped into thinking that every research statement must be right. The period of research will also enable them to approach the unanswered questions in day-to-day work in a much more enlightened and acceptable way.

5. It is never possible to prove unquestionably any hypotheses, but well-conducted unbiased experiments will allow statements to be made about the probability of their results being valid.

2. When, what, where, and supervision

Overview

An individual attracted by the idea of research, needs to get down to the practicalities of: assessing its advantages with regard to a future career; when to do it, where to go, what to research, and how to gain funds. This chapter sets out the main considerations in making these decisions. It also details the role and responsibility of the supervisor, and emphasizes the researcher's need for self-discipline and motivation.

When to undertake research?

The need for, and timing of, a period of research in a career programme, is usually laid down within the traditions of each speciality. It is generally at a postgraduate level, by which time the candidate has a basic knowledge and insight into the boundaries and limitation of the field. In many fields the initial research period comes directly after an undergraduate programme. In the medical field there is usually an intervening service commitment of 1–5 years. This separation should generally be as short as possible, since research experience can be a valuable asset when undertaking subsequent appointments. Once the decision to undertake a research position has been taken, it should preferably be in a full-time capacity so that commitment can be total. This is not to decry undertaking part-time research in any intervening period, but try to ensure that any work of this nature is under the guidance of an experienced individual, and follow the suggestions laid down in this chapter. Research is not an easy option, it takes time, effort, and money. Occasionally a candidate takes on such a position at a reduced salary and this highlights the need to have specified goals and a precise time schedule. Whereas a 6–9 months apprenticeship provides some indication of what postgraduate research is about, to undertake, complete and write up a piece of work in the form of a thesis takes at least two, and preferably three, years. The regulation of most postgraduate degrees state the expected time schedule.

Whether an individual stays on in a research position is partly decided by the personal satisfaction gained and partly by career and financial implications. Long-term research still needs at least two full days per week, is approximately 40 per cent of the workers time, to allow continuity of the practical elements, and time to think and discuss an ongoing programme. Subsequent appointments and progress are related to the success of an initial research period. A wider experience must then be obtained in the field; a 3–5 year period abroad is often a valuable addition to a training programme. It takes 8–12 years to gain international recognition in a field, most researchers being established by the age of 35–40. They can then command appropriate support from grant-giving bodies and hold secure positions in universities and in industry. Although the headship of a department provides a certain autonomy, it also carries with it many time-consuming management tasks, the demands of supervision, completing of grant applications, and administration. These responsibilities take the research worker away from practical aspects of everyday research; careful thought must therefore be given before accepting such positions too early in a research career. The reward of such an appointment is related to directing a research team, rather than individual involvement, and must be accepted as such.

What field, where, and how funded?

Research is undertaken on a specific topic chosen from a wider field of interest. An inexperienced worker commencing a period of full-time research must join an institution researching in the chosen field, even if it means moving to another region or spending some time abroad. On no account should an inexperienced researcher attempt full-time research in isolation. If the field of study is undecided, the beginner should keep an open mind and consider one or more departments working in an area appropriate to a future career. The main essential is to join a unit where research is being actively undertaken and where expert help is assured. Such a unit will usually provide the multidisciplinary team approach, so essential to present-day research, and the possibility of collaborative involvement and training in all aspects of a research programme. A well-equipped department will also provide the beginner with desk space, computer facilities, time and expertise, appropriate apparatus, and technical help. Within these confines examine more than one department and, if possible, a different one from that attended for the first degree. This will provide an alternative approach to a subject, widening the interest and approach to the field. All these factors, however, are dependent on availability and the competition for appointments. Before visiting a department to discuss a research position be sure to be acquainted with the research carried out within it. Read its current publications, abstracts of presentations to learned societies, and theses, examining both their quantity and quality. Particularly examine activity in the chosen field of interest, and determine the number of staff, research workers, and students in training. Discussions with members of the department will indicate the likely direction of any subsequent research. Enquire as to the entitlements of postgraduate students, with regards to supervision, facilities, technical, and secretarial help, and out of hours access to buildings. Look at the style of working of a department. Talk to the likely supervisor and other members of the department, both staff and students, to assess whether it is appropriate. Examine the code of practice of the department, the interdependence of its members, the freedom to discuss ideas, and whether regular meetings and discussion groups exist. Assess how a new student will fit into this pattern and whether they are allowed freedom and flexibility within a team, or whether they are just a part of a research factory. From the publications, work out who makes the presentation at learned societies and who takes senior authorship of published material. Research is a highly competitive field and the department ground rules should be determined before taking up a post. Admission to a department is usually dependent on obtaining an appropriate class of degree or other qualification and previous experience. Appointment is usually after an interview with the head of department and one or more members of staff, including the proposed supervisor. There may be an initial probationary period, or registration for a masters degree prior to showing satisfactory progress and going on to a doctorate. All these factors should be discussed, agreed, and placed in writing prior to acceptance of a position. An active university department and laboratory may have adequate resources for research assistants, scholarships, and junior lectureships, or the offer of a position may be linked with the acquisition of money from government bodies, trust funds, foundations, or drug companies. Grant applications are a critical form of research presentation and are considered in Chapter 20.

The length of the research appointment may be related to the money available or the university requirement for a specific degree. A 2 year or preferably a 3 year period is usual. Some appointments are linked with a moderate or heavy clinical or teaching commitment; this is undesirable as it will slow down the rate of progress of the research project. Such commitments often detract from the research, particularly if the project is passing through an initial frustrating period.

The foregoing comments are not intended to discourage commencing a research interest on a part-time basis, but a clear distinction should be made between this type of project and one which has to be completed within a set period for a post-graduate award. Experienced workers may have to combine research and teaching appointments, but even this can only be achieved by the strict discipline of maintaining set times in the laboratory, particularly if a substantial part of the time is spent in clinical teaching or administration. Experienced workers will have technicians available to help them. For the inexperienced worker it is important to carry out the procedures personally: this is mandatory when preparing for a higher degree.

The topic

The topic on which the research project is to be developed must be decided as soon as is feasible. Consideration has already been given to the choice of field, this being linked with the student's interests and with the choice of department. The student will discuss a specific topic with the head of department and proposed supervisor before commencing an appointment. This must now be developed into a clear question with a proposed answer. Advice from supervisor and other experienced research workers is essential at this stage, as an inappropriate choice of topic is likely to spell disaster for a project from its outset. Many pitfalls exist and experienced personnel can prevent a student from wasting time. Thus the project must be agreed with the supervisor and senior members of staff prior to its commencement, and be within the policies, capabilities, expertise, facilities, resources, available equipment and cost boundaries of the department. In this way staff members will continue taking an active interest and involvement, and will be able to comment and help if progress at any time is unsatisfactory. The topic must be of sufficient scientific merit and interest to warrant investigation, and also be of an appropriate depth of study to satisfy the proposed degree. It must be original or, if previously undertaken, there must be a good reason for repeating the study: new knowledge and techniques can throw a different light on previous investigation, presenting a reasonable chance of finding something original. The choice of topic must present a practical proposition. Although novel topics are desirable and exciting, they are not necessarily rewarding and generally it is better to choose a topic where an outcome is assured, even if a negative result is obtained. Ideas and proposed solutions must be viable: they must not be too difficult or impossible, and must be within the capabilities, and appropriate to the skills and understanding, of the student. Simple concepts are best, with clearly defined and circumscribed objectives. The magnitude of the task must be such that it can be completed in the allocated time with a reasonable chance of success, and without overwhelming an inexperienced researcher. The tasks must not be too complex, but sufficiently detailed to demonstrate the ability of the student to carry out and complete a research project. In the case of human experiments requiring patients, their availability and ethical consideration must be carefully thought through in advance.

To a newcomer the choice of research topic is often daunting and in practice most workers at this stage in their career have no firm ideas. However, in the majority of scientific fields hard data is scant and many questions are available for detailed examination. Be on the look-out in the literature for gaps, inconsistencies, areas of uncertainty, questions, unexpected findings, suggestions, alternative explanations, unsubstantiated claims, unqualified statements, and speculation. A broadly based topic may have several lines of development and it is useful to start with two; this provides an escape route if one aspect comes to a dead end at an early stage of development. One of the major advantages of a large laboratory is that a student can be involved in more than one aspect of a topic. At all times, however, remember that the award of a postgraduate degree is based on a student's personal originality, planning, and development and, therefore, must be based on independent activity.

The supervisor

After joining an active research team the first essential is to find a suitable supervisor (precentor). A supervisor should be a full-time member of staff, actively involved in the same field and be available throughout the proposed research period. The choice is usually related to the topic and there may be no alternatives. On the rare occasions when the supervisor is not a member of the department, a full-time member of staff should be nominated who will be responsible for the student's progress, since this ultimately rests with the department concerned. If a supervisor takes sabbatical leave or undertakes a lengthy overseas trip, consideration should be given to a replacement or introducing a supplementary advisor. This should also be the case if a supervisor has a period of illness. The head of department or the postgraduate tutor should have regular meetings with both supervisor and student, and may be in a position to fill in this back-up role. The number of students any one member of staff should be supervising must be small and within their capabilities with regards to experience, and other teaching and administrative duties. Close matching of personality and interests of the supervisor and research worker is highly desirable as incompatibility can spell disaster to the future of the project. If a gross mismatch is obvious before commencing, alternative arrangements should be carefully considered. There should be a clear mutual understanding of the respective responsibilities of the supervisor and student, preferably written down prior to the start of a project. The researcher may not have much say in their form of supervision, but the rest of this chapter is intended to provide them with some insight into the problems of supervision and what they should expect of a supervisor. Departments should have a document available to student and supervisor, laying down its views on good supervisory practice.

Role and responsibilities of the supervisor

Supervising a student who is pursuing a postgraduate qualification is not necessarily a rewarding task. The supervisor may not have chosen the role or the student, but does have the responsibility of bringing the research to completion. The rules, regulation and the standards of the proposed degree must be known, ensuring that the student does so as well. The supervisor will be closely involved in the choice of topic and will monitor progress throughout.

The amount of involvement by a supervisor in a research project can vary from active participation to peripheral surveillance of progress. Involvement is usually maximum at the outset of a research programme, when the supervisor explains the nature of research and is involved in the planning of the project, and laying out a timetable of events and requirements. If a clear time schedule is not laid down and adhered to at the beginning of a project, each stage is likely to get further and further behind. At this stage a student requires a good deal of guidance in how to read around and effectively study the field: the supervisor must identify gaps of knowledge, understanding, and technical skills. In planning the research programme a naive student may have little insight into the feasibility or practicability of procedures, or how long they will take. Ethical codes of practice and departmental policy may have to be considered and the whole fashioned into a balanced programme or work. Progress is more assured if a student joins an ongoing project, but in this situation the supervisor has to ensure that the student does not just become another pair of hands, but has ample opportunity to exercise original thought. Simply analysing data without involvement in the development of a project, regardless of the amount of work undertaken, will not in itself be enough to satisfy the requirements of a higher degree. The extent to which a student is trained in each aspect of the project, or is thrown in at the `deep end', should be related to the student's temperament and ability.

The supervisor should be aware of a student's attendance record and progress in all aspects of the agreed programme, encouraging and maintaining impetus throughout. Meetings should take place at least weekly in the initial phase. The supervisor should receive regular written progress reports and review essays during the course of the work, as well as encourage publication in suitable journals, once meaningful data is available. These preliminary writings will greatly simplify the eventual writing of a thesis. Regular assessment, including tutorials, mock vivas, checking experimental records, and maintenance of a time schedule, is particularly relevant if the student has been taken on for an initial probation period. Presentations at departmental seminars should be organized to obtain constructive critisism, particularly prior to presenting any material to learned societies. Feedback from the supervisor should indicate the quality of progress to the student, the likely outcome of the project, and identify areas requiring modification or improvement. The supervisor should provide regular written reports on the trainee's progress to the head of the department. At the end of the first year it is advisable to do a formal assessment of a trainee's performance. This may include written work produced during the year and/or a clearly identified piece of work written specifically for this occasion. The assessment should be by the supervisor and another expert, and include a viva examination. In this way an objective report can be made, the trainee receives appropriate feedback and a work plan can be formulated for subsequent stages. It will ensure that the student is suitable to continue with the project and that the project itself is likely to yield an outcome in the allotted time. If there is doubt about the latter, at this stage, it is still possible to change to a topic which can be completed on schedule. The supervisor should ensure that complete and systematic records are kept of all aspects of the research. Examination of this material will ensure it is available for writing up at a later stage, that it is appropriate to the needs of the project, it also demonstrates the understanding of the project by the trainee. The records should be such that the research could be repeated or unfinished areas reinvestigated at a later date from easily defined outlines. The supervisor should see the first draft of each section of a thesis, although the final format, discussion, and conclusions are very much the responsibility of the student.

Another possible requirement of a supervisor is to take part in the oral examination of a thesis. The main task is to help the student feel relaxed and provide the external assessors with clear background information. The supervisor should not become personally involved in any arguments with an external assessor.

Student responsibilities

As soon as a student has decided to prepare for a postgraduate research degree the regulations from the university registrar should be obtained. These have to be adhered to precisely and registration undertaken promptly, as a university does not usually allow retrospective work to count against the regulated research period for the degree. Even if the title of the thesis has not been finalized the provisional title should be registered as this can be modified at a later date. Generally it is better for the student to ask for help and make it clear how much supervision is mutually acceptable. Frank regular discussion is essential. The student should attend regular meetings with the supervisor and bring along current problems. It is the student's responsibility to maintain progress and produce verbal and written presentations to an agreed time schedule. The final draft of a thesis is totally the responsibility of the student.

Student/supervisor relationship

If at any time during the research a supervisor feels the student is putting in inadequate time or effort, or lacks the necessary ability to complete the project, this must be discussed with the student. If this fails to resolve the situation, the facts should be placed in writing and a dated and signed copy placed with the university registrar. The department should monitor progress of both student and supervisor at research committee meetings. There should be a mechanism for changing a supervisor in the event of total incompatibility and this should be done without loss of time, money, or face. Usually, however, the relationship between student and supervisor is a respected and lasting one, and the initial apprenticeship often culminates in a partnership of research into a mutual field of interest.

Summary

1. The timing of a higher research degree depends on the field of interest but it should be undertaken as soon as possible after the primary degree.

2. Whether this first period of research proves to be a satisfying experience depends to a large extent on where the individual goes. An extended visit is essential to find out about styles of work, facilities offered to students, and arrangements for supervision.

3. The supervisor–student relationship is a close and important one, and discussions with a prospective supervisor are critical.

4. The supervisor has a responsibility to ensure that a student receives training in all aspects of a research programme and completes a research project in the alloted time.

3. Literature review, action plan, and pilot study

Overview

Setting off on a research programme can be a time of great uncertainty and indecision, as well as excitement. A topic will have been chosen but the problem to be studied may still be rather vague and the means of answering it even more ill-defined. At this stage the researcher needs to proceed along two pathways. The first is to undertake a great deal of reading and, linked with this information gathering, to set up a storage system as considered in the following paragraphs. The second pathway is to create an action plan for the research project; this is considered on p. 23. The importance of clear planning, and the common lack of it in failure to complete a postgraduate degree, is emphasized by the concern of universities and scientific bodies, many of which have laid down codes of practice. These documents also consider the level of attainment required by examining bodies and the student should read carefully those pertinent to their field of study.

Reading plan

The awareness of the time taken to read and digest a single article, when attempting to gain a brief acquaintance with an unfamiliar scientific field, leaves the new researcher in no doubt as to the need for a selective choice of reading matter. Reading has been said to rot the mind, and certainly 1–2 months intense, but disorganized or arbitrary reading of a new subject can leave the uninitiated confused and lacking any clear ideas of the basic components of the topic. First read a general textbook and then a specific textbook or monograph on the subject. There follows a search for leading articles and reviews, which will lay down basic principles and identify prime references in the field. Trace those articles which are most frequently mentioned and emphasized in the reviews. Eventually all articles quoted should be read and not just quoted from a second source. The advice of a supervisor or experienced worker in the field should be sought as to the main papers which should be read during the initial planning of the project. The searches of the literature obtained can be gradually assimilated during the course of the research, together with the relevant papers from current specialist journals. The journal of the chosen specialty must be thoroughly examined each week or month, since this will also be the target journal for subsequent reporting. The journal will also contain invited commentaries, letters, reports on relevant meetings, and leading articles on associated topics. When writing up the literature review of a thesis, at a later stage in a research programme, all relevant literature must be comprehensively covered. This includes video material, dissertations, theses, reports of congresses and conferences, and reports on specific research meetings, possibly published by industrial companies.

Literature catalogue

In spite of the much quoted information explosion of the last two decades, and of the startling figures as to the number of scientific journals and articles now in existence, computer science has remained abreast of the problems, and the scientist has available clearly defined methods of retrieving the information pertinent to his or her field of interest. A lot of research time is spent in the library and at the commencement of a research programme the uninitiated should seek the help of a skilled librarian. The librarian will indicate the layout of the building and position of the appropriate books, journals, and catalogues. The librarian will also provide computer searches into specific aspects of topics, on- or off-line, and update this essential information as often as requested. This is usually obtainable at a reasonable cost, but the researcher should also become fully conversant with all computer searching systems available in the library, where they can do their own searches. Other services that are usually available include, tracing and obtaining articles from the library, or other libraries by interlibrary loans, and photocopying facilities. Librarians differ in their methods of classification and cataloguing and it is important to understand the local system with regards to shelf and room markings and codings. Catalogues indicate the works held, together with subjects, titles, and authors, and any missing numbers of a journal series.

Most developed contries have a national library which has by law to obtain copies of all writings of that country, together with a number of specified foreign works. These include The National Library in London, The National Congress Library in the US and the French Bibliotheque Nationale. However, access to these specific libraries may be difficult for a trainee and there are many excellent alternatives. In the UK, in addition to university libraries, the libraries of learned societies, of the Royal Colleges, and the National Lending Library are such examples.

Scientific and medical literature is generally well organized. One of the most comprehensive interdisciplinary indexes is the *Index Medicus*, available in all good scientific libraries. It is published monthly and contains medical, nursing, and dental literature published throughout the world. Over 2500 journals are included and articles are usually referenced within 3 months of publication. Classification is by both author and subject and foreign language articles are identified; the index contains a section on review articles and this indicates the number of references included. *Index Medicus* forms the basis of many of the computer retrieval systems discussed below. The researcher, however, needs to have clearly and closely formulated subject headings when searching in the index, in order to obtain only articles of specific interest and not to be overwhelmed with inappropriate material. Each January a new volume of medical subject headings and codes (MeSH) is published to use with *Index Medicus*, indicating new and obsolete terms. The number of indexes is expanding to match specific scientific needs and their format and the benefits of each should be discussed with the librarian. *Excerpta Medica*, for instance, is a quarterly publication listing journals (approximately 3500), books, and conferences. It is more extensive in its cover of medical literature than *Index Medicus*, but some references may take a year to be included. *Biological Abstracts* covers clearly defined experimental, medical, and life sciences, giving brief summaries of articles from specified journals. Abstracts of articles in foreign languages are included and are very useful as translation can be very expensive. When using *Biological Abstracts*, all possible key words, together with their plurals and adjectives, must be considered to ensure maximum retrieval of relevant information. *Chemical Abstracts* provide a valuable means of accessing this area of literature. *Current Contents* is a weekly issue of the contents of specified journals. It provides the researcher with rapid access to titles which could otherwise take many months to retrieve. Further indexes, such as the *Science Citation Index*, list the papers that have cited key references, leading the researcher into a variety of associated fields in a very specific way. Be on the look-out for indexes specific to your field of interest, as these are more likely to cover the totality of any field. Examples are to be found in psychiatry, kidney disease and nephrology, health care administration and health care management.

Computer information searching

Computers are widely used in research to simplify the task of searching the literature. This, otherwise, can be very time consuming and is prone to error, inadequate retrieval, and expensive duplication of material. An initial examination of *Index Medicus* and other indexes provides the researcher with experience of what is available and to know how information is stored. Browsing also sends the researcher into many interesting and alternative channels. However, once this type of experience has been obtained, there are many more efficient and effective ways of reviewing the available literature. In the last 15 years on-line information searching has developed to such an extent that linking up to a database is very easily achieved. The first thing to be decided is the selection of the appropriate database (category of journal). This will usually be a computer searchable version of a standard indexing system such as the Cumulative Medical Index. The Medical Literature Analysis and Retrieval Service (MEDLARS) set up in the early 1960s was an early attempt to automate searches from *Index Medicus* and the current version of the system (MEDLINE), is a highly sophisticated means of searching the literature. A hard disc with a database extending back to 1966 is available in most libraries. This CD-ROM (read only memory) is updated monthly and contains a tutorial programme for training in its use; abstracting indexes are available in similar form. The information can be obtained by the use of key words from the terms in a thesaurus and these facts can be printed out or transferred onto floppy discs for use on a microcomputer. The Article Delivery Over On-line Information System (Adonnis) covers

219 biomedical journals commencing in 1987 and individual articles can be accessed on-line. The most complete database has been developed in relation to Aids, which is the Compact Library Aids and incorporates compact disc references from all available sources. The seriousness of the disease and its comparatively recent discovery have stimulated the need for, and facilitated the comprehensive nature of, the index. Equivalent databases on other diseases are currently appearing.

The researcher must learn how to access and retrieve data through the on-line facilities. Begin the search with either a specific term or with a more global one such as 'hypertension' and then narrow this to a more specific phrase, for example hypertension in endocrine disease. The work of a specific author may be requested or citations of a specific paper. Limits may be imposed, such as English language papers only or a specific time period, for example 1978–1982. The output received varies on request, from brief details such as author, title, bibliographic citation, to a comprehensive abstract or printout of the full article. These facilities are now widely obtainable and provide a thorough means of performing a literature search and save a great amount of a researcher's time.

Information storage by the researcher

Start classifying all collected materials, and all ideas formulated, at the outset of a research programme. The process of amassing information is continuous through-out research and it is vital to assemble these facts in an orderly fashion. This cataloguing can be done in various ways and should be guided by both librarian and supervisor. Start a file of references, coded alphabetically by the surname of the first author. Wordprocessors and appropriate software are now widely available and allow new references to be added to a list in alphabetical order; as well as cross referenced by subject and other chosen groupings. These facilities have largely out-dated the card system of cataloguing, although this is still an efficient system where suitable hardware is not available. Every reference system should contain the names and initials of all the authors, the year of publication, the full title of the paper, the name of the journal, the volume number, the first and last page numbers, and the source of the reference. Most scientific journals now follow the Vancouver system of referencing, and punctuation can follow this scheme (p. 190) with one exception: although the Vancouver system reduces the number of authors to a maximum of seven, all names must be included in the researcher's catalogue. These reference lists provide valuable sources of material for future presentations: researchers vary in the amount of information about a publication they transfer onto a computer. It is advisable to retain photocopies of each article when this facility is available, highlighting important facts and sentences for future rapid retrieval.

Collect reprints, photocopies, and other relevant information in subject folders, each representing a particular aspect of the project. New articles are added to subject folders sequentially and given a number that can be recorded in the refer-ence system, with a code indicating that the material is available. As the number of articles accumulates, folders will give way to filing cabinets but meticulous labelling and filling is the key to efficient running of all systems. Once a filing system has been established all material can be stored and none lost or wasted. Key words can be used for subclassifying references and allow retrieval of specified groups of publications: a well-organized filing system, containing full and accurate information, can save a large amount of time when writing papers at a later date.

Critical reading

When reading a paper start with a detailed examination of its abstract or summary. The introduction provides a few useful sentences about the topic, but this will soon become repetitive after examining a number of papers on the same subjects. Approach the methods and materials, the form of analysis and the results critically, examining every statement and determining whether they are relevant and appropriate to what is being examined. Remember that just because something has been published does not mean that it is right, neither is a statement right just because it has been written by an eminent person. Beware the 'opinionated fact', i.e. something that has been generally accepted but is based on opinions which have never been tested. The discussions section of a paper provides ideas on many important questions still unanswered and places the findings in a wider context. Ensure that the conclusions are justified by the methods and results. In particular, look for gaps, inconsistencies, unsubstantiated claims, speculations, unexplained and serendipitous findings. At the end of reading an article, write down a few comments on its methodology and its conclusions, and an opinion on its value. Key phrases may be taken down to be quoted later, but for the most part it is better to convert this information into one or more carefully written paragraphs and to store this on your computer database. These summary paragraphs can be used in this form or in modified fashion when writing papers or a thesis at a later date.

Action plan

The researcher should spend a few days writing a comprehensive *protocol* or *action plan* as soon as the topic has been chosen and preliminary reading has started. This should follow the headings laid down in the next section and these will act as the framework on which to build the whole research programme. The protocol should end up as a typed, dated, and numbered discussion document for consideration by the supervisor and all members of the team who are going to be involved in the research projects. It will also serve as a basis for discussion with other experts who may be involved directly or peripherally with the study, such as clinicians or statisticians. It does much to clarify ideas and highlights matters of feasibility, resource implications and ethical considerations. The document can be started and roughed out and some sections written during early reading and enquiry: it must be completed and discussed before commencing the practical aspect of the programme. If necessary, the same material can be used as the basis of a grant application.

Headings for the action plan

1. *Title*. This should be between three and eight words long and contain the key words relative to the project. A subtitle of 5–10 words may also be needed for more precise definition of the field.

2. *Aims of the study*. Start the section with a sentence stating the aim of the research. If this requires more than one sentence it is probable that the experimental design includes too many factors, and the subsequent results will almost certainly be meaningless. The question for which a solution is being sought must be clearly defined. If the aim is too complicated it may also be difficult to complete the study in a limited time.

3. *Background of the field*. This is a historical review of 500/600 words containing 6–12 relevant references, numbered in order of presentation and quoted in the final section. The review indicates the background of the field and the events leading up to the need for the study, written in a logical sequence. It finishes with the proposed solution to the problem indicating why this is likely to be a productive line of investigation.

4. *Methods and materials*. This section is the most detailed part of the protocol. The plan of the investigation must be given in full. This may be by surveying naturally occurring events or by manipulating events in a controlled fashion. These factors are considered in Section B and advice may be needed from experts, such as an epidemiologist or statistician. Remember that the validity of the results is entirely dependent on the use of an appropriate statistical design: the methodology of both design and analysis must be decided *before* the commencement of the project. The number of groups and subgroups should be kept to the minimum necessary for valid results and full consideration given to the choice of subjects. Above all the influence of any factor not rigorously controlled must be entirely free from bias. The proposed technique should include operative details, and whether *in vitro* or *in vivo* experiments are to be used, also details of dosage and frequency of administration of drugs, chemicals, radiopharmaceuticals and anaesthesia, together with operative details of any surgical procedures. The apparatus required should be listed, together with its availability. The safety implications of the project must be outlined (Chapter 7). Specify how data is to be collected, measured, analysed, presented, and interpreted. References must be given for the documented techniques being used, and numbered sequentially after those from the review. If human subjects are being used for a particular investigation or a therapeutic trial, outline the proposed groups and indicate the number of individuals that are thought to be necessary in each. The ethics and responsibilities in human investigations are considered in Chapter 5. When animals studies are planned a number of other factors must be considered. The species of animal used depends to some extent on the facilities available, the number of animals required, their availability and their cost. More important, however, is the suitability of the animal for the procedure to be undertaken. The ethics and responsibilities in animal investigations are considered in Chapter 6. Animal licences may take a number of months to process so they must be applied for as soon as possible in a research programme. They are further considered on p. 44.

5. *Organization*. The place where the investigation is to take place must be stated and the names of all participants and collaborators listed (with their consent). State when the study is to commence, how long it is to last, whether it will be in stages and, if so, the times scheduled for each part. List the facilities available and those required, including technical and secretarial help. State areas where further expert help will be required.

6. *Finance*. The financial implications of a research project will be unknown to most new research students, however, early training in this area is essential: no institution can ignore the financial implications of research projects being undertaken within their precincts. The cost of the project with regards to its capital and running costs should be outlined, together with hidden costs, such as the use of existing laboratories, libraries, computer facilities, and technical and secretarial help. Other expenses may include travel of researchers and subjects.

7. *References*. A numbered list of full references should be included matching those cited in the text.

Discussion of the action plan

The protocol should be discussed fully with the supervisor, who, from previous experience, will be able to point out defects and will probably suggest some modification of the programme. In collaborative work the responsibilities of each investigator must be agreed and documented. At this stage it is also wise to discuss the order of authorship in any subsequent reports, a matter considered in more detail on p. 185. If human or animal subjects are involved in the study, the protocol is also assessed by an independent ethical committee. The latter's principal function is to prevent pain, discomfort, and harm to individuals and it is particularly concerned with the use of radioactive and hazardous substances. Ethical committees and their responsibilities are discussed in Chapter 5. The ethical committee may well advise modification of the protocol or request further information after a pilot study. Once these comments have been obtained the protocol should be modified and the next version dated and numbered, circulated to participants, and, where requested, resubmitted or discussed with the ethical committee, before proceeding to the practical stages of the project.

Pilot study

A pilot study must be undertaken prior to commencing the full investigation, in order to assess the feasibility and practicability of the research design, and to ensure that the investigation as laid out in the protocol is realistic. It also indicates the number of measurements that will be needed to provide meaningful results. The size of response and subject variation will be identified, together with the appropriateness of the control measures. Temporary or borrowed apparatus can be used for a pilot experiment, but the availability of the appropriate apparatus for the definitive study must also be assured. If animal surgery is planned, preliminary post-mortem anatomical studies must be carried out to gain familiarity with an operative procedure. The pilot study often identifies unexpected problems requiring modification of the protocol, such as an inappropriate choice of animal and failure of a piece of apparatus or of methodology to meet reported claims. The efficient running of all aspects of the protocol, therefore, must be assured before proceeding. On completion of these preliminary observations, appropriate modification is made to the research protocol and a further (possibly final) version prepared with clearly defined goals and deadlines. This must be re-presented to the supervisor and collaborators and may require further approval from the ethical committee. After these various stages the definitive investigation can commence.

Use of time

Setting up these experiments may take a number of months and is likely to encounter many setbacks and delays. The frustration of this initial phase is known to all research workers, but make use of any spare time to improve knowledge in any subjects in which there has been inadequate prior training. Common examples are found in areas of computer technology, statistics, electronics, radiobiology, and immunology. Essays on specific topics provide important training for writing papers and theses. Keep a *diary* of proposed and completed activities, as this stimulates, reassures and forms a basis for discussion with the supervisor: *it is an essential component of all research programmes*. This is also an ideal time for further information gathering and the period can be used to visit other centres with specific interest and experience in the field. Be continually on the look-out for new ideas and for unanswered questions on the subject appearing in the literature or in discussion with other workers. At all stages of the research take every opportunity to discuss the project with members of the department. In this way a comprehensive knowledge of research activities is acquired and it will form an excellent grounding for a future research career, be this in an experimental or an applied branch of science. Getting started and completing a pilot study usually takes 6–9 months of a 2 or 3 year project.

Summary

1. Having successfully chosen a research department, selected a suitable problem and completed the background reading, success is within grasp—providing the remaining time is used to good effect.

2. Organized reading at this stage is essential. This is an active and exacting task in which notes are taken and records kept of relevant material. It is from this reading that ideas emerge as to the questions that need investigating.

3. An action plan is needed. This sets out the problem to be examined. Time is allocated to all aspects, including pilot work and the final writing of the thesis. Discussion with the supervisor is essential before implementing the action plan.

4. Undertaking and completing a research project

Overview

The basic training has been completed and the larger part of the reading around the topic has been undertaken. The topic has been selected and a pilot study will have demonstrated the feasibility of the methods, the reliability of the apparatus and the probability of success. The division of the work between collaborators should also have been sorted out. What now remains are the stages of data collection and analysis, followed by reporting the result in papers and theses.

Data collection

This phase is a period of active investigation during which the bulk of data collection takes place. It is generally the most enjoyable, as, in spite of long hours of work, the efforts are rewarded by the acummulation of results and the early frustrations are over. The bulk of the formal training is over and the topic refined. The researcher will also have developed good practices of time keeping and be able to lay down his or her own schedule of target completion dates. Data must be collected in an unbiased, organized, reliable, and comprehensive manner: hard-backed books rather than scraps of paper are used and, when not in use, stored in a secure place. Precise documentation and tight security are essential in human and animal experiments, where there is a legal as well as a moral requirement for doing so. Careful consideration must be given to the use of computers to store data and, when they are used, security must be assured. Data stored in this way can be rapidly available for analysis at any stage of the study. Computers, however, are subject to breakdown, loss of data, delay in access, time-consuming programming and expense: back-up hand written results must always be available and kept until analysis is complete. Advice should be sought on the use, abuse, and limitations of computers in data storage, from an expert in this field. This phase of experimentation takes one-half to two-thirds of the allotted period of research time. Time scheduling and sticking to a planned programme are still necessary. The period must not be allowed to extend into the time set aside for writing up at the end of the project. The major reason for not completing a research project is failure to write up the study, rather than noncompletion of the practical components. It is often difficult to know when to stop and there is a strong tendency to go off at tangents; this tendency must be avoided as the arbitrary following of interesting lines is fatal to the completion of any proposed thesis. A single-minded approach is essential to complete a project in the prescribed time. Discussions with the supervisor must identify any additional work necessary before bringing investigations to a halt.

As the data is collected preliminary analysis is undertaken, setting out the results in graphs and tables to indicate trends and unexpected findings. This information may be used to modify the investigations. However, any change should only be carried out in conjunction with the supervisor and the statistician involved in the original research design, since certain designs do not allow for major changes. Results should also be continually monitored and regularly discussed with the supervisor and senior colleagues in order to prevent excess accumulation of data. Stockpiling unexamined results is a certain pathway to failure. It is also possible to get distracted at this stage in over-analysis, getting hooked on computer technology. Individual results requiring extensive analysis must be handled as they occur: discrepancies may be easily explained and if necessary sorted out if identified early. Care however, must be taken that 'knowledge' of some results does not bias future collection of data. It will be possible to complete the format and content of most tables towards the end of the phase, together with the illustrations of the methods and apparatus. Methods and results of completed sections can be written up during this phase and reading must be kept up-to-date with detailed cataloguing of references. The review section of a thesis can also be largely completed in this phase, writing out the developments in the field in a chronological order and in a critical manner. Write on large sheets of paper using wide lines or alternate lines so that alterations can be easily undertaken. As preliminary results become available they should be presented at departmental seminars. These discussions will clarify the likely number of results required and can modify the direction of activity, thus avoiding excessive data collection and loss of direction. As hard data becomes available it can be presented to a wider audience and research societies. It is also helpful to arrange a mock viva on the work, while there is still time to undertake additional reading and a further limited amount of experimentation.

Completing the thesis

Completing a project within a set period of time can be very difficult for an experienced research worker and it is therefore not surprising that a large number of students fail to complete a project in the prescribed time. The pitfalls of getting started have been emphasized, some of these, such as unexplained findings and difficulty in making apparatus function satisfactorily, may be unavoidable. Of probably more importance, however, is the discipline required in the middle phase of a research programme, when collecting data. A definite time schedule must be adhered to. Reporting research findings is of equal importance to completing the experiment: it is an integral part of research experience and a researcher's responsibility to the funding body. Writing a thesis is also one aspect of a project which is the total responsibility of the student. Time must be allowed within the research period for completing the writing, since taking up another appointment inevitably puts a complete stop to this activity. Internal promotion within a research department should be, and often is, conditional on submission of a thesis to the examining body; moves to another position should be discouraged until a thesis has been submitted. The prospect of financial rewards, while appealing, must be restrained, since such a move will dramatically slow the writing of the thesis and may stop it completely, possibly to the long-term detriment of promotion. The distribution of the workload in the 4–6 months required to complete a thesis is considered in a later section (p. 198). Keeping to a fixed schedule is difficult and the use of a diary to plan target dates for each section and to check progress is essential. Writing can be slow even for an experienced researcher and may appear insurmountable to the beginner. The supervisor should again take an active role in this campaign. Inadequate supervision results in more than half the titles submitted for a thesis in some fields not being completed within 5 years. Reasons for failure are various: some candidates have great difficulty in completing anything, others get overburdened with masses of literature and data, and cannot see the wood from the trees, while others are never satisfied with the outcome. It is the responsibility of the supervisor to identify these problems and guide and support the student through difficulties. Students in turn must give total commitment to the project, question each step and set themselves achievable goals. A well-planned and disciplined research project will ensure that the time spent is both productive and enjoyable.

Summary

1. Data collection is one of the most satisfying parts of a research project but it must be kept within a strict schedule and data analysed as it is produced. If there are continual slippages in the time schedule, the activity that will suffer most is the final one, the writing of the thesis. Without a thesis there can be no higher degree, no matter how well the research was undertaken.

2. An important part of the discipline of research is to record what was done with sufficient accuracy and detail that somebody else can repeat the work and test the findings.

3. The whole point of research is to further knowledge and understanding, and this requires dissemination of the results.

5. Biomedical research on human subjects

Overview

Medical progress is based on research which, ultimately, must rest on experimentation involving live human subjects. Most societies prefer animal in preference to human experimentation, but results from the former are not always applicable to the latter. The use of animals in research is considered in Chapter 6: this chapter considers the ethics of human experimentation. The purpose of biomedical research is to improve the understanding of the structure and function of the body in health and disease, and test the effectiveness of various ways of diagnosing, treating, and preventing disease. Clinicians must at all times only act in the interest of the subject, whose health must be their first consideration. Before deciding to carry out a research technique, therefore, they must take account of any hazards of an experiment to the subject, such as a drug side-effect. They must also draw a fundamental distinction between research where any benefit is directed at the subject, and research in which there is no direct benefit to the subject. Essential guidelines for clinicians undertaking biomedical research on human subjects are provided by the declaration adopted by the World Medical Assembly in Helsinki in 1964, and modified in 1975 and 1983. Researchers must also take into account the legal requirements and the recommendations of professional bodies in their own country, and formulate their own ethical opinions and obligations to their society. In the UK additional information has been published by the Department of Health[1] and the Royal College of Physicians of London.[2] One of the recommendations of the Helsinki declaration was that specially appointed committees should receive the experimental protocols of all procedures involving human subjects. In many countries ethical committees already exist to consider, comment on, and give guidance on research projects involving human subjects. The following paragraphs consider the structure and function of an ethical committee and the general principles that they, and the research worker, should consider.

Ethical committees—structure and function

Institutions undertaking research on living subjects, fetal material, and the recently dead should have an ethical committee. The committee provides informed medical and lay opinions on the range of research topics submitted and is free to co-opt members to discuss difficult and sensitive areas. Members of the committee should be elected by responsible authorities and act on the committee as individuals. The scientific representatives must command the technical competence and judgement to assess the physical, mental, and personality consequences of the proposed research and the majority should be actively involved in clinical care. In the UK, therefore, the representatives may comprise: a hospital clinician, an individual experienced in clinical investigation, a general practitioner, and a practising clinical nurse. Lay members represent community interests and must be of appropriate responsibility and standing in the community, and not be overawed by the weight of scientific opinion. Frequently, they have a legal background since this can be helpful in assessing and balancing statements and ideas. Both sexes are usually well represented. Members of the committee who have personal interests in any submission, must declare it and normally do not take part in this discussion. The purpose of the ethical committee is to facilitate good biomedical research in the interest of science. Members will question and discuss ethical issues, accepting that there may be no single correct answer and that codes of practice will change in time and place. The committee must preserve the rights of the subject and protect them from possible harm, working in the public interest in establishing the highest ethical standards for all research in its institution. The committee will also protect the research worker from any unjustified attack. Much of the work may be covered in committee and this has the advantage of mutual exchange of views; material is distributed beforehand. Applications of minor ethical concern can be managed by the chair's action; all such action is reviewed later by the committee and accurate records kept of all decisions. The number of meetings will depend on the work load.

Submission to the ethical committee

The investigator is expected to submit details on all research (undertaken at an institution) on living subjects, fetal material, and the recently dead. Optional policies, leaving the decision as to what raises ethical questions to the investigator, defeats the purpose of the committee. The ethical principles, which should be considered by the investigator and the ethical committee before the research is undertaken, are set out later in this chapter. The importance of distinguishing between research which is of benefit to the subject (therapeutic research) and that which is of no direct benefit and carried out on volunteers (nontherapeutic research), has already been emphasized; in the case of nontherapeutic research, changes to the subject must always be of a temporary nature. Ethical approval may be required even when the research does not interfere with the subject, as when case records are examined. In the UK the Data Protection Act relates to all human personal details in record departments on computer. EC laws, aimed at unifying data publication across Europe, may increase the restrictions on researchers, particularly with respect to epidemiological analysis. The administration of drugs and undertaking procedures for educational purposes, such as in the training of doctors, should also be subject to approval of a local ethical committee. Research into the effects of drugs form an important aspect of biomedical research. This research is subject to the general ethical principles aready outlined, as well as requiring the submission of additional information to the committee: the information required is set out later in this chapter. The committee should see all advertisements for volunteers and copies of the consent form. Research in obtaining tissues from the recently dead should ensure the application of internationally accepted criteria of death. Cadaver organ transplants must be in accordance with the laws of the country where the organs are being donated. The special considerations of live donor transplantation to be taken into account by the investigator and the ethical committee are set out below. In the UK, reference 1 provides useful guidelines for ethical committees and research workers in this area. The majority of projects examined by an ethical committee will involve participation of consenting adults and the committee will require evidence that the subjects are being fully informed not only of the details of the project but also of their individual rights. In minor procedures, which entail minimal discomfort or inconvenience, such as withdrawing an extra volume of blood, obtaining consent may cause unnecessary distress and the committee may consider it reasonable to proceed without it. Research involving children and those incapacitated by intellect, culture, and mental or physical disability or disease, require detailed consideration. In all these cases consent must be obtained from the legal guardian or a responsible relative; in some cases this is obtained in addition to the consent of the subject. Examples of consent for different categories of subject are provided below. New and novel methods of diagnosis or treatment introduced in patient management and for the benefit of patients, are usually subject to the ethics of a doctor - patient relationship, rather than an ethical committee. When incorporated into in research project they may become so. If a clinician or researcher is in any doubt as to whether a project requires ethical approval, he or she should always communicate with the chair of the ethical committee by letter or word of mouth.

An ethical committee should give directions on the format of each submission or provide a standard application form. This will ensure that information is obtained on all debatable issues: the standard format will save committee time. A committee should also see all advertisements for volunteers and copies of proposed consent forms. The confidentiality of all materials considered by the ethical committee must be honoured by its members, in order to maintain the standing of the committee in the community.

Decisions

While total rejection of a project is rare, the committee may refuse applications on grounds of inadequate scientific quality. It is unethical to submit subjects to potentially harmful yet fruitless research projects which are badly designed or will not produce meaningful results. It is common for projects to be modified after discussion with an ethical committee. If the committee considers certain aspects to be weak it may suggest seeking expert advice in these areas. The onus is always on the applicant to satisfy the requirements of the ethical committee. If a project is turned down the reasons should be given to the applicant in writing and if the decision is challenged it may be appropriate to appoint an arbitrator acceptable to both sides. Although ethical committees are not usually able to apply sanctions to unheeded advice on projects which have or have not been submitted, failure of an investigator to comply with local ethical committee requirements, is likely to incur sanctions from the governing body.

Monitoring

While it is desirable for an ethical committee to monitor the progress of all research projects of which it has approved, this may be impractical. It may, however, request a periodic report on each project and follow specific controversial projects in more detail. The reports and publications on all approved projects should be received by the ethical committee; all reports and publications should indicate that the research has received the committee's approval. The committee should be informed of all adverse experimental effects occurring in its institution.

It is the responsibility of the committee to keep itself up-to-date with current published literature on ethical matters and all such material should be distributed to each member.

Multicentre trials should normally be submitted to the ethical committee of each institution involved. This may be cumbersome and give rise to different opinions. Ideally, therefore, participating centres should agree on a single ethical committee, either set up by the organizers of the trial or an independent professional body. Unfortunately this is not always possible.

Key points

1. Clinicians at all times should only act in the interest of the subject whose health must be his or her first consideration.

2. Ethical committees help the researcher to meet his or her commitment to the subject, by:
    (a) Having as their first consideration the physical, mental, and psychological interests of subjects.
    (b) Providing medical and lay opinions on ethical issues.
    (c) Assessing the technical competence, and judging whether research projects are well-designed and capable of producing meaningful results.
    (d) Protecting the investigator against unjustified criticism.

3. Investigators are expected to submit to the ethical committee all research on living subjects, fetal material, and the recently dead. Even when the subject is not being interfered with, there may be a need to submit a project to the ethical committee, as when case records are to be examined.

4. Advice should be available to the researcher as to the format required by the ethical committee in submitting a proposal for a research project. Besides taking into account the general principles of research on human subjects, the ethical committee will be looking for the researcher to have taken specific note of requirements when using drugs, cadaver organs and live donor transplants, and fetal material.

5. The ethical committee will also want to see copies of the consent forms used, together with all advertisements for volunteers. For subjects too ill, too incapacitated, or too young to understand the meaning of giving consent, a legal guardian or responsible relative should be asked in place of, or in addition to, the subject.

General principles of research on human subjects

1. The research should represent a justifiable advancement in biomedical knowledge that is in keeping with the prevailing community interests and priorities.

2. Research must comply with generally accepted scientific principles and should be based on a thorough knowledge of the scientific literature.

3. Human research must only be undertaken after comprehensive experiments, and then only if these experiments do not provide all required information.

4. The research should not take place unless the hazards involved are believed to be predictable. Preliminary laboratory and animal experiments must be sufficient for assessment and definition of these risks and inconveniences. Risks should be compared with the foreseeable benefits to the subject and others, and the research should not be carried out unless the importance of the objective is in proportion to the inherent risks to the subject. The study must cease if hazards are found to outweigh potential benefits.

5. The research must have minimal impact on the subject's physical state, mental integrity, and personality. The interests of the subject must always prevail over the interests of science and society.

6. The privacy of the subject and all data generated by the research must be respected. The confidentiality of data generated by the research must be ensured, particularly when it can be attributed to an individual subject. The information on all research data must be stored in locked cupboards in secure rooms and accessed on a system of file only by designated individuals. Where possible, names and data should be stored separately and identifiable data must not be transmitted across public communication lines. Anonymity must be maintained in published results.

7. Each subject must be adequately informed of the aims, methods, anticipated benefits and potential risks of the study, and the discomfort and inconvenience it may entail.

8. The subject must be at liberty to abstain from participation and at any time free to withdraw without reason. Withdrawal must not influence subsequent management, incur displeasure, or give rise to questioning.

9. Freely given informed consent should be obtained, preferably in writing Consent forms should be written in simple language, incorporating the factors outlined in paragraphs 7 and 8. The form used should be approved by the ethical committee and signed by a witness ascertaining that the consent had been freely given and fully understood. The form should be retained for a statutory period of not less than 6 years by the principal investigator or, in the case of a patient, after an initial 6-months period, in the case records. Formal consent in no way reduces the responsibility of the investigator and it does not remove the ordinary rights of the subject.

10. In case of legal incompetence (physical and mental incapacity, and minors) informed consent should be obtained from the legal guardian or responsible relative in accordance with national legislation. Whenever a child is in fact able to give consent, that consent must be obtained in addition to consent of the minor's legal guardian. For further advice on research in this group of patients the reader is advised to refer to reference 2.

11. The proposal should include a statement of ethical considerations and indicate how these principles have been complied with. A protocol should be submitted to an ethical committee, together with all consent forms and advertisements and couched in a language which is easily understandable to a layman as well as to a scientist.

12. The design of the experiment should be clearly formulated and likely to achieve its proposed objective. The project should have been discussed with experienced clinical scientists who can identify errors and inadequacies.

13. The minimal number of subjects compatible with the satisfactory completion of the study must be used.

14. Appropriate facilities must be available to carry out and complete the research programme.

15. The research should only be carried out by appropriately qualified and experienced personnel; the responsibility of the human subjects must always rest with medically qualified personnel and must be approved by the clinician in charge of their overall care.

16. Distinction must be drawn between research carried out on patients for their benefit and nontherapeutic research on volunteers (whether healthy or patient volunteers) without direct benefit to the subject (see below).

17. Particular attention must be given to dependent relationships, such as patient volunteers, and consent must not be obtained under duress. If possible, informed consent should be obtained by clinicians not involved in the research and independent of the official clinical relationship.

18. Nursing staff should be made aware of any research in progress on patients under their care and of ethical committee approval.

19. The question of payment of subjects should not arise in therapeutic research but volunteers should be compensated for their out-of-pocket expenses and possibly

for risks, discomfort, and inconvenience. Ethical committees should be informed of the level of payment and be satisfied that it in itself is not primarily an inducement to become involved. Acceptance of payment should in no way impair the ethical and legal rights of any subject. Commercial organizations not infrequently pay an institution to test new drugs and appliances. In its consideration of such projects selected members, or under certain circumstances all members, of an ethical committee should be aware of the extent of such support and whether it is a direct cash transaction or payment of salaries, equipment, or other expenses. Information should also be disclosed about whether any member of the team is a paid advisor to the company concerned.

20. The accuracy of results should be preserved in publications and ethical principles upheld. It is an editor's responsibility to withhold publication if these principles are not achieved.

Therapeutic research

1. A clinician must be free to use new diagnostic and therapeutic measures if in his or her judgement it offers hope of saving life, re-establishing health or alleviating suffering.

2. Potential benefits, risks, and inconveniences of a new method should be weighed against those of the best diagnostic and therapeutic methods available.

3. In a trial, every patient, including those of a control group, must be assured of the best proven diagnostic and therapeutic methods.

4. Refusal of a patient's participation in a research project must never interfere with a clinician–patient relationship.

5. If a clinician considers it essential not to obtain informed consent, this should be stated in the experimental protocol submitted to an ethical committee.

6. Combining research with medical care is only acceptable if it is of potential diagnostic or therapeutic advantage to the patient.

Research on volunteers

1. It is the duty of the clinician to protect life and health of the research subject at all times.

2. Except in extremely minor procedures, informed consent of the subject should be obtained in writing as well as verbally.

3. If volunteers are recruited from an institution their responsible officer, for example dean or works medical officer, should be informed of the details of the research and any proposed payment, together with the ethical committee's approval of the project and advertising methods. Adequate time should be allowed for approval of each volunteer by the responsible officer.

4. Recruitment of volunteers in institutions is best undertaken in group situations or notices rather than by a direct individual approach.

5. The subject must be questioned on current or recent involvement in other studies which could influence the outcome of the research. The problem of research on volunteers is also considered in Chapters 12 and 13.

Drugs

1. This research is subject to the general ethical principles already outlined. Preliminary laboratory and animal studies and full toxicological data must be available therefore to an ethical committee.

2. National regulations vary considerably in this field. In the UK medicines can be classified as follows:

(a) Marketed drugs which have a product licence—there is little difficulty in the use of these drugs in controlled experiments and in investigations on newly found properties.

(b) With new products the producer lodges a proposal with a licensing authority. This is administered by the Medical Division of the Department of Health and where appropriate is issued with a clinical trial certificate (CTC) or an exemption from the need of such a certificate (CTE).

(c) When a product is imported and has no UK pharmaceutical agent or is a chemical, the investigator may apply to the licensing authority for a CTC.

(d) Studies on drugs on healthy volunteers do not at present require any form of licensing (but do require the agreement of an ethical committee).

3. Investigators must state the classification of all drugs in their application to an ethical committee and provide a summary of the toxicology and all known properties. The existence of a CTC or a CTE does not mean that the drug or the research project have been adequately reviewed and does not diminish the responsibility of the investigator to get approval of the ethical committee.

4. The committee can only make any judgement on the information supplied and, if this is insufficient with regard to data about the drug to approve a research project, they may suggest a more limited study followed by reappraisal.

5. The committee will consider what arrangements have been made for compensation to a subject in the event of an injury, independent of any proven fault. The Association of the British Pharmaceutical Industry (ABPI) has laid down guidelines on medically induced injuries.[3] In the case of premarketing drug studies instituted or sponsored by an industrial company, a written statement must be obtained from the company that it accepts these guidelines. Unsponsored research on premarketed drugs or any research on drugs with a product licence does not usually have the same insurance.

6. Drug effects or injuries incurred as a result of research in the UK can only be compensated legally if negligence can be proven on the part of the research worker. Responsible research organizations and the Department of Health have stated that they may offer *ex gratia* payments to volunteers injured as a result of participation

in clinical investigations. Nevertheless it is often difficult to establish a causative relationship between the disability and the research, and payments are likely to be made without any admission of liability. Ethical committees thus carry a high responsibility in ensuring that subjects are adequately protected, and will look extremely carefully at the research application.

7. The use of radiopharmaceuticals are well controlled in most countries where they are in routine use. In the research situation care must be taken to exclude volunteers whose work does, or is likely to, involve contact with any form of radiation, so that they are not over exposed.

8. Drug research also raises the ethics of the use of the placebo. When a placebo is administered, or effective treatment is otherwise withheld, the investigator must justify these intentions to an ethical committee. If effective treatment is available, a more satisfactory approach is to test a new product against the best available treatment. Even when effective measures are available, however, a placebo is sometimes necessary as part of the experimental design, when subjects improve without any drugs. It is usual to tell a patient that at some time during treatment an inactive drug will be administered with the intention of distinguishing between imaginary and real effects of treatment. In these circumstances the ethical committee will be particularly concerned to check the adequacy of continuous subject monitoring independent of whether a trial is single- or double-blind in its format.

9. Only in exceptional circumstances should a patient not be informed that they are in a trial situation (for example in the management of a terminal illness) and this decision must be incorporated into the submission to an ethical committee.

Live donor transplantation

Although the ethics of transplantation are predominantly those concerning a doctor–patient relationship rather than ones involving an ethical committee, a number of ethical problems do exist. Cadaver organ transplants must be in accordance with the laws of the country where the organs are being donated. A live donor transplantation is more controversial. The benefits of the transplant to the recipient are considerable. In the case of renal transplantation, for example, improved health and a dialysis-free existence. The benefits to a donor are less tangible and the risks not negligible. A live kidney donation is only justified if there is a shortage of cadaver organs. Transplantation from a blood-related donor offers a good chance of success but the relationship must be confirmed if necessary by using DNA finger printing. The best match is between identical twins, followed by siblings and parents. The satisfaction of helping a child or sibling can not be denied but the relationship gives rise to the possibility of family pressures. The relation must be totally without coercion. Whereas it might be unethical to totally exclude unrelated donors, such transplants should only be undertaken in exceptional circumstances, applying rigorous safeguards and satisfying rigid criteria in order to avoid exploitation of donors or the manipulation of recipients, and to afford adequate protection for doctors. The following list is not exhaustive and items may change, it will however serve as an initial guide in the field.

1. The donor must have reached the age of legal majority.

2. Unrelated donors should be limited to a spouse or a friend whose close and enduring relationship can be established beyond doubt, if necessary by appropriate documentation.

3. The consent for donation must be freely given and the motivation must be altruistic and charitable. There must be no monetary transaction other than reasonable expenses and reimbursement of loss of earnings.

4. The offer of donation must not be in response to any form of advertising and gaining publicity must not be a motivating factor.

5. There must be no family or other pressure, blackmail, or extortion involved.

6. The donor must be sufficiently informed and conversant with the attendant risks, including preoperative angiography, the surgery, possible complications, potential financial losses, and insurance liabilities.

7. It should be emphasized that there is no guarantee that transplantation will be successful.

8. The donor must be of mature and emotionally stable character. A psychiatric assessment is advisable.

9. The donor must of sound physical health. If there is any disparity of the function between the two kidneys, the poorer one should be transplanted.

10. The social, family, and other commitments and obligations of the donor must be taken into consideration.

11. Until these various problems have been fully discussed and informed consent has been freely given the recipient should not be party to this discussion and the donor must be left a possible outlet such as on the grounds of tissue incompatibility.

12. The procedure should only be undertaken by recognized fully equipped units with extensive cadaver transplant experience, thus ensuring full investigation, excluding adverse factors and increasing the likelihood of a successful outcome.

13. The confidentiality of donor and recipient must be respected at all times.

In the UK the British Transplantation Society has recommended the setting up of a government-sponsored review panel to register all organ donations and transplants and documenting all importation and exportation of donor organs.

Sample form for submitting a research project to an ethical committee

1. Title of study.

2. Summary of project (100–150 words).

3. Aims of study.
4. Background of project.
5. Plan of investigation, place of study, anticipated timing and expected duration.
6. Methodology ((a)–(h)).
   (a) Subjects—proposed numbers.
       (i) Patients (enclose copy of consent form).
           Adults.
           Children.
       (ii) Volunteers—(enclose proposed consent form: the names of students and volunteers from institutions will require approval by their responsible officer before involvement). Patients—Source: university, institution.
       (iii) Method of recruitment (enclose any proposed advertisement).
       (iv) Proposed reimbursement and fees.
       (v) Methods being taken to ensure confidentiality of personalised data.
   (b) Techniques.
       (i) Collection of blood, other body fluids, excreta or tissues (state amounts).
       (ii) Invasive techniques.
       (iii) Non invasive techniques.
   (c) Risks, discomfort, and inconvenience involved and measures taken to minimize these.
   (d) Experience of the applicants in the field of the investigation.
   (e) Design of the experiment
   (f) Method of collection and analysis of data.
   (g) Reliability of results.
   (h) Drugs and licensing status (p. 37)
       (i) Product licence.
       (ii) CTC or CTE (attached copy).
       (iii) CTC applied for.
       (iv) Healthy volunteer study—no application made.
       (v) State if letters of indemnity have been obtained from the sponsor to cover any injury to patients or volunteers (enclose copy).
7. Payment from sponsor or related concerns (financial details to be forwarded separately to chair of ethical committee—financial details will normally only be known to the chair and one lay member of the committee),
   (a) Will any investigator receive any personal fees or rewards in respect of this study?
   (b) Has the department or any related department received any financial contribution from the sponsor over the last 3 years, or is any anticipated?

(c) Have any of the investigators or their immediate associates ever acted as a paid advisor to the sponsor?

8. Names and signatures of the chief investigator and all investigators and collaborators in the study.

9. Name and signature of approval of any consultant who is in charge of patients in the study and is not included under paragraph 8.

The completed form, consent form, advertisements and an appropriate number of copies, together with a separate financial statement, should be forwarded to the chair of the ethical committee by the stated date for consideration at the next meeting.

Sample patient's consent form

Consultant ....

Investigator ....

Purpose of study and description of study to be carried out.

I understand what this study involves and I agree to take part in it on the understanding that refusal will not affect my treatment in any way and that I may withdraw at any time without question.

Signature of patient ....

Full name ....

Address ....

....

Date ....

I have been present while the procedure has been explained to the patient and I have witnessed his/her consent to take part.

Signature of witness ....

Date ....

(the witness should *not* be connected with the study.)

Statement of consent of healthy volunteer, whether student from an institution or other source

In understand what this study involves and agree to take part in it on the understanding that I may withdraw at any time without question.

State the research studies that you have been involved in the last 3 months (if none write 'none'). [I understand that my responsible officer—(dean, works medical officer) is aware of the nature of the study, the dates it will be undertaken and of my informed participation.]

Statement of consent for child under 12 (over 12)

I understand what this study involves and agree that my child should take part on the understanding that refusal in no way affects my child's treatment and that he/she may withdraw at any time without question.

(I have had this study explained to me and I agree to take part in it; additional signature of child over 12 years).

Summary

1. The ultimate aim of biomedical research in humans is to improve their physical and mental well-being. Experiments should only by carried out on humans when progress can no longer be furthered through examination of previous work or research on animals. Before deciding to go ahead with research on humans, the balance of benefits and risks must be carefully considered. This is particularly so when nontherapeutic research is carried out on volunteers.

2. Research on humans includes fetal material and the recently dead, as well as living subjects. The definition also includes research where individuals are not interfered with, but information about them investigated.

3. The primary means by which the interest of individuals are safeguarded from unethical research is the ethical committee. Such committees are concerned with the efficiency of the proposed research design as well as direct consideration of its ethics. It is unethical to submit subjects to possible harm when the poor design of an experiment will lead to meaningless results or more subjects are being used than are needed to reach a conclusion.

4. Besides full details of the proposed investigation, the ethical committee will require to see copies of advertisements if volunteers are to be used, together with copies of proposed consent forms. Consent should normally be obtained from subjects, or, when necessary, the legal guardian or responsible relative. It is not for the researcher to judge whether a piece of research on living subjects, fetal material, or the recently dead should go before the ethical committee—it is for the ethical committee to make a judgement about whether there are aspects of the research requiring their consideration.

5. Individual patient management, involving untried methods of diagnosis or treatment, is subject to the ethics of a doctor–patient relationship, rather than an ethical committee. As soon as the method of diagnosis or treatment is investigated further

through a research project, it becomes the concern of an ethical committee. If in doubt, the matter should be raised with the chair of the ethical committee.

6. Guidelines for carrying out biomedical research on humans are listed above; a distinction is made between therapeutic research on patients and nontherapeutic research on volunteers. Special considerations should be taken into account when researching into the effects of drugs.

7. Research in obtaining tissues from the recently dead should be in accordance with internationally accepted criteria for death. Cadaver organ transplants must be in accordance with the laws of the country where the organs are being donated and transplanted. Reference 1 sets out the main issues relevant to research in this area.

8. Having approved a project, it is likely that an ethical committee will wish to monitor its progress in some way.

9. Besides protecting subjects, an ethical committee also protects the researcher from unjustified criticism.

References

1. Department of Health (1972). *The use of foetuses and fetal material for research*. HMSO, London.
2. Royal College of Physicians of London (1984). *Guidelines on the practice of ethics committees in medical research*. RCP, London.
3. Association of the British Pharmaceutical Industry (1991). *Clinical Trial Compensation Guidelines*. ABPI, London.

6. Biomedical research on animals

Overview

It is a matter of great public concern that the use of living animals for scientific procedures should be limited to the minimum compatible with the pursuit of legitimate scientific ends. Statistical advice should be obtained to achieve this objective, and adequate consideration given to the feasibility of obtaining the same information by means not involving the use of animals. It is one of the general principles of the Council of Europe Convention on the protection of vertebrate animals used for experimental and other scientific purposes, that nonsentient alternatives to animals should be used whenever practicable. All successful methods of study which can refrain from the use of animals should be publicized and published. When no alternative is available to the use of animals, the researcher must be guided at all times by the principles of humane and meticulous experimentation, and a sense of moral as well as legal responsibility for an animal's welfare, throughout the time it is cared for.

Legislation in the UK

In the UK, the legislation relating to animals is incorporated in the Animals (Scientific Procedures) Act 1986 which came into operation on 1 January 1987, replacing the Cruelty to Animals Act 1876 with a new system of control on scientific work. The A(SP) Act of 1986 provides for the licensing of experiments or other scientific procedures applied to a *protected animal*, which may have the effect of causing that animal pain, suffering, distress, or lasting harm. Such work is referred to in the Act as a *regulated procedure*. Protected animals are defined as all living vertebrate animals except man; the definition extends to fetal, larval, and embryonic forms which have reached specified stages in their development. Under the Act an animal is regarded as living until the permanent cessation of circulation or the destruction of its brain, thus procedures carried out on decerebrate animals are subject to its controls. The controls do not extend to procedures applied to animals in the course of a recognized veterinary, agricultural, or animal husbandry practice. There are certain other exceptions such as ringing, tagging, and marking animals for the sole purpose of identification.

Under the Act licensing is required of *premises*, *projects*, and *personnel* concerned with protected animals. The type of animal, the purpose of the procedure, the procedure itself, and the type of technique are coded for subsequent analysis by the Home Office: licensees are required to keep records and project-licence holders make annual returns of these details to the Home Office. The Home Secretary is required to lay before Parliament guidance on: the operation of the controls, the codes of practice as to the care and accommodation of animals, their use in scientific procedures, and the collection of annual statistics. Major offenses against the Act carry penalties of fines and imprisonment and breaches of the conditions of licensing may result in revocation of such licences. The Act gives statutory recognition to the Home Office Inspectorate to give advice and assistance to licensees and other personnel.

Designation of premises. Any place where work is carried out under the Act must be designated as a scientific procedure establishment by a certificate issued by the Home Secretary. In addition, establishments which breed certain types of animal for use in scientific procedures, and establishments which obtain such animals for elsewhere and supply them to laboratories, must be designated by a certificate. All designated establishments are inspected by the Home Office Inspectorate and will be required to nominate a person to be responsible for the day-to-day care of animals: a veterinary surgeon must be available to advise on their health and welfare.

Personal and project licences. Two kinds of licence are required for all scientific work controlled by the Act. The person applying the regulated procedure must hold a *personal licence*, but in addition the procedure must be part of a programme of work authorized by a *project licence*. No work may be undertaken unless the procedures, the animals used, and the place where the work is carried out, are specifically authorized by both personal and project licences.

Personal licence

A personal licence is the Home Secretary's endorsement of the holder's competence and suitability to carry out specified procedures on specified animals. Applicants must be over 18, and submit their qualifications, training, and experience. Normally they should possess the equivalent of at least 5 'O' levels or have received appropriate formal vocational training. Many licensees will be subject to a condition of supervision, this normally remaining in force for one year. Undergraduate licensees remain under supervision until they have completed their degree course. Project-licence holders have a general responsibility to ensure that personal licensees working on a project carry out their work properly and humanely, and keep within the terms of the project licence. Imposed supervision, however, in no way lessens the individual responsibility of the licensee to comply with the provisions of the Act and the terms and conditions of the licence. A personal licence is normally granted for an indefinite period, but is subject to review at periods not exceeding 5 years. Licences for undergraduate students are subject to annual review. The licence should describe the location of the work and be amended as required. The purpose of the procedure, the type of animal, and the technique must be detailed in an application, as discussed in subsequent paragraphs. If the applicant has not previously held a licence, has not been resident in the UK for the past 5 years, or has not enough understanding of English as a native language, a sponsor is required; the sponsor is normally a senior scientist in the department in which the licensed work is to be carried out. The sponsor is expected to provide assurance on the applicant's competency, character, and understanding of the law. Personal-licence holders are responsible for the welfare of all protected animals under their care. He or she must clearly label cages to enable identification of the project, the responsible licensee and the principal procedure. It may be most appropriate to code the procedure, but this information must be easily obtainable by the inspectorate.

Project licence

A project licence will be granted when the Home Office Inspectorate considers that the use of live animals in a programme of work, is justified and the methods proposed appropriate. In deciding whether and on what terms to authorize the project, the Inspectorate is required to weigh the likely adverse affects on the animals used against the benefits likely to accrue from the work. The Inspectorate must also be satisfied that the applicant has adequately considered the feasibility of using alternative methods not involving live animals. The holder of the project licence must be someone who undertakes full responsibility for all scientific direction of the work. This will generally be the senior personal licensee engaged in the project. The project-licence holder must maintain records, in the form approved by the Home Office, of all animals on which procedures have been carried out under the authority of the project-licence. Each January the project-licence holder has a statutory obligation to complete statistical forms of all procedures commenced during the previous year and return them to the Home Office. The returns must include information of change of name and change of professional address or place of work. If the licensee ceases to conduct regulated procedures on living animals for the foreseeable future, or decides to leave the UK for more than 3 months, the licence should be returned to the Home Office. Returns are addressed to Room 976, Home Office, Queen Anne's Gate, London, SW1H 9AT.

Involvement of unlicensed persons in animal experimentation

It is quite permissable for an unlicensed technician to feed and care for animals during a scientific procedure, but a licensee can not delegate tasks such as dosing or collecting blood samples, since these would be considered procedures likely to result in pain. Assistance in holding and restraining animals can be given by unlicensed persons, who can also help the licensee in carrying out surgical procedures. Although there is a fine distinction between helping and carrying out a procedure, it is a useful practical rule that a licensee should always be present and physically involved during the period in which scientific procedures are being carried out.

Records

Records must be kept for each protected animal and retained for a 5-year period following the death of the animal. These records should include: the source, the species, the breed or strain, identification (individual or batch), date of arrival, where bred (on site or date of transfer), approximate age on arrival, sex, whether pregnant, date in and out of quarantine or isolation, microbiological status (gnotobiotic, SPF or conventional), harmful genetic defects, and project licence to which allocated. Records should include the name of the project-licence holder, the deputy project-licence holder (where applicable), project-licence number, and the names of personal licensees involved. Details of procedures should include: the species of the protected animals used, the number of each species used, the sex and approximate age at commencement of the regulated procedures, the date of commencement of the regulated procedures, any unexpected morbidity and mortality, brief description of procedures, any reuse within the project, the date of the end of the regulated procedures and the fate of the animal at the end of the regulated procedures (whether released to the wild, dispatched to private care, released for slaughter, killed within the establishment or, if permission for reuse was granted, identification of the project to which the animal was allocated).

Each animal must be readily identifiable. In the case of dogs, cats, and primates this must be by an approved method of permanent marking; other protected animals should bear a label stating: the cage or area identification, the animal's individual or batch identification and the date of arrival. A health record relating to protected animals must be kept at the designated establishment, under the control of a veterinary surgeon or other suitably qualified named person. All records have to be available for examination by an inspector at any time.

Assessment of applications

All applications for licences and certificates are considered by the Home Office Inspectorate who recommend whether, and on what terms, the application should be granted. External assessment of part or all the application may be required; particularly for highly specialized research and novel techniques. The applicant will be informed if an outside assessor is consulted. The assessor will be an expert from an invited panel covering the main branches of the biological sciences. The final decision rests with the Home Secretary. Applications may also be referred for advice to the Animals Procedures Committee, as will all applications for work on cosmetics, on conscious animals involving tobacco products, and for training in microsurgery. The Animals Procedures Committee was established as an advisory body, to have regard to both the legitimate requirements of science and industry, and the protection of animals against avoidable suffering and unnecessary use in scientific procedures. Personal licences and certificates may be granted with appropriate conditions attached, and the Act empowers the charging of fees. A person whose application for authority under the Act is refused or whose licence or certificate is to be revoked or varied, other than at their own request, has the right to make representations to an independent legally qualified advisor appointed by the Home Secretary. The advisor will consider any representations and the Home Secretary will take the advisor's view into account when making a final decision. The checks and safeguards involved in the granting of a licence are time-consuming. This is particularly so when novel procedures are involved or where an applicant has given insufficient personal information, or information about the project. These factors must be taken into account when applying for a licence, since no one may carry out a regulated procedure until the appropriate authority of a licence has been obtained. Further information, such as lists of protected animals and the procedures that can be undertaken, can be obtained from Animals (Scientific Procedures) Inspectorate, Home Office, Queen Anne's Gate, London, SW1H 9AT. Biomedical trainees undertaking research outside the UK should contact national governing bodies for information concerning animal research in their country. Researchers should be aware of these regulations even if not personally undertaking any animal experiments.

Summary

1. In the UK the Animals (Scientific Procedures) Act 1986 governs the use of animals in research. This can be used as a useful guideline for researchers in other countries as to an accepted standard. Alternatives to animals should be used whenever practical.

2. Under the Act premises, projects, and personnel involved in the use of animals in research must be licensed.

3. The project-licence holder is required to send annual animal returns to the Home Office indicating the number of animals used, their status, the form of anaesthesia, and the type of procedure being investigated.

4. Biomedical research workers outside the UK should be aware of their own national regulations concerning animal experimentation.

7. Health and safety in research

Overview

The observation of routine safety precautions is very much a part of modern life. Such measures are even more important in a laboratory environment, where the potential hazards of mechanical and electrical equipment, and chemical, biological, and radiation materials may be present. All new recruits must have made available to them copies of an institute's statement of policy which, in the UK are legal requirements under the Health and Safety at Work Act.[1] They should also have identified to them the safety officer of the institution and the department safety officer and be informed of the codes of practice in operation in the institution, and given guidance on safe practices. Many universities hold introductory and specialized courses on safety for its personnel and all individuals should attend these as soon as possible after appointment. Individuals should be signed up as having attended such courses and also sign that they have received and understood this information. Education must also be extended to domestic staff who clean laboratories as to where they can freely go and any precautions needed.

Laboratory accidents should be minimized by the good design of the area and the apparatus used but it is only after thorough training of personnel in laboratory safety and with continued supervision that the important commodity of common sense can be expected to take over. The ultimate responsibility for the safety of individuals in a laboratory, be they academic or nonacademic staff, postgraduate or undergraduate students, research workers or members of the public lawfully entering the precinct, rests with the governing body of the institution. However, employees have a duty to take reasonable care to avoid injury to themselves and others, and ensure optimal care and safety for all animals under their jurisdiction. The researcher should examine the attention given to health and safety when first assessing an institution as this is one of the factors indicating the quality of its activities. Similar concern must be given to setting up and carrying out every research programme. An individual contemplating a new area of research should write down the procedures proposed, set out possible hazards and communicate with the safety officer and the safety committee before commencing. It is essential that descriptions of procedures should be kept up-to-date. This chapter is intended to provide preliminary guidance on safety, and alert the research worker to potential dangers that may be encountered.

Statutory regulations and the function of the safety committee

Health and safety in a research environment in the UK is governed by the Health and Safety at Work Act 1974,[1] and regulations subsequently made under the Act and coming into operation in 1978. These regulations advise that the governing body of a laboratory, be it a university or research institute should set up a safety committee and appoint a safety advisor. Further subcommittees and departmental officers should be appointed in relation to requirements. The composition of a safety committee should reflect the interests of the institution, all departments being represented particularly those of microbiology and those using ionizing radiation. Provisions were also made under the Act for recognized and independent trade unions to demand the establishment of a safety committee, if this had not already been undertaken. The function of a committee and its officers can be considered under the headings of policy making, education and implementation, and safety monitoring.

Policy making

The statement of policy of an institution should contain the essence of the employer's approach to safety and indicate the line of responsibility from the governing body down to each individual. The safety committee should be conversant with existing local and national literature on safety procedures, such as the local code of practice in a university and the Department of Health code of practice on ionization radiation. It should supplement this advice with rules pertinent to local circumstances compiling its own local code of safety practice. These rules do not necessarily constitute statutory legislation on safety, but allow for the differing nature and purpose of the work. Legislation itself is of course unable to compel observation, but can only penalize failure and the purpose of both systems should be to prevent injury, and subsequent legal proceedings being an unfortunate consequence of failure. The committee should recommend and advise on policy, and changes of rules, to both the governing body and to all personnel. It should maintain a close liaison between other connected authorities, such as local government officers, fire departments and police departments, when circumstances require.

Education and implementation of safety procedures

It is the duty of the safety committee to ensure that all personnel are taught relevant safety precautions. In large institutions this education may be delegated to specialist subcommittees such as mechanical and electrical, chemical, biological and radiation protection. Any booklets should be circulated on publication and each new member of the institution should receive all relevant material and instruction. Practical instruction should be given on all potentially hazardous procedures followed by supervision until they are mastered. Untrained personnel, particularly, must not be allowed to handle heavy machinery, high voltage appliances, or dangerous chemical, biological and radioactive material. The safety officer in most institutions is an amateur rather than a professional and works in an advisory capacity to the governing body of the institution and the heads of departments. It is the duty of the safety officer to put up appropriately sited and relevant warning signs and instigate regular training sessions, such as fire drills and the use of fire-fighting equipment.

Safety monitoring

The safety committee and its officers should ensure that the standards of safety that they have proposed and taught should be maintained and this part of their duty above all other, requires continued vigilance and periodic spot checks. Safety measures should become an attitude of mind at any institution and be part of everyone's routine. Repeated checks should be kept on the monitoring of film badges, first-aid facilities, alarm systems, and fire-fighting equipment, ensuring that emergency exists and corridors always allow access and fire doors are not fixed with wedges or by other means. If an occupational health service is available it should be involved in both assessing and controlling hazards. Regular medical checks may also be indicated when the possibility of contamination with harmful materials exist. Clear records in hardback books or as filed reports should be kept of all accidents or incidents with precise details of the incident, the facts being carefully sought in the form of written, dated *and* signed statement from the injured person and observers. The safety officer and safety committee should be notified of all such incidents. In the UK reporting of injuries, disease, and dangerous occurrences (near misses) during work is mandatory following the Riddor report of 1985. This initially is by a telephone call, within 24 hours, to the local representative of the Health and Safety Executive, followed by a written report within 7 days. Any accident that prevents an individual from carrying out ordinary work for greater than 3 days is included. Some of the most important aspects of safety are the handling, storage, and disposal of harmful products. The following paragraphs provide some guidelines in these matters, together with advice on handling electrical and heavy appliances. The safety officer should identify and label hazards, hazard areas, and all containers of harmful products, using the appropriate signs. Examples are flammable, explosive, toxic, corrosive, compressed gas, and radiation (radiofrequency, microwaves, infrared, ultraviolet, lasers and ionizing radiation, such as X-rays and radiotherapy).

Handling of harmful products

There should be adequate room for storage of such material away from working areas and public throughways, and waste disposal should have strict local rules, based upon local and legal requirements. Hazards include explosive, corrosive, inflammable or toxic chemicals, biological material, infected animals, harmful bacteria and radioactive substances.

The design of laboratories using dangerous products should allow adequate room, wide unobstructed corridors, automatic doors, and large flat continuous working areas which can be cleaned easily and decontaminated. Flooring also should be easily cleaned and be of the nonslip variety. If wet processes are used there should be suitable drainage, and personnel should have appropriate footwear. Lighting should be good, even if windows, for reasons of security, privacy, or construction, are limited; no movement of these materials should be undertaken in the dark. Good ventilation is necessary, as are controlled temperature and humidity, the air being replaced at least 6–10 times per hour. Fume chambers may be required and occasionally some form of respirator used when gaseous and volatile toxic materials are being handled.

Storage areas should generally be close at hand (an exception being with inflammable products), since this allows dangerous substances to be transported only short distances to the laboratory. Stairways and other obstructions should be avoided and corridors kept clear; automatic doors are useful. Storage areas should be locked and all products should be meticulously labelled. The quantities of dangerous products being stored and used should, where possible, be the minimum compatible with effective laboratory usage. Storage areas must be at the appropriate conditions to avoid dangerous changes to occur of the stored contents.

Electrical facilities

Laboratory services must be expertly installed and all apparatus designed with safety in mind. Electrical apparatus must be handled and checked by trained personnel with particular reference to fusing, circuit breakers, earthing and insulation. Leads should be of the correct length, i.e. not too short or leaving a dangerous trailing length. Any apparatus constructed in a department must be subject to the same stringent requirements of electrical safety and checked by trained personnel at the time of installation and all appliances checked at 3–4 monthly intervals. Generally all apparatus should be turned off at the end of a working day. When it is necessary to leave certain appliances on continuously, such as ovens and fridges, signs to that effect should be marked over the switch controlling the apparatus.

Electrical hazards include burns and shocks. It is unusual to receive a dangerous electrical shock from less than a 120 V source. When inflammatory material is being handled potential sources of ignition such as smoking, flames, electrical, static, hot materials, and ovens should be eradicated. Cold rooms should have doors which can be operated from both sides and alarm systems installed. All defective appliances should be labelled as such and removed from service until faults have been rectified.

Light, noise, and vibration

Some laboratories may require ultraviolet or infrared light sources or laser apparatus. Shielding must then be effective and exposure of personnel avoided. Those working in the vicinity of such apparatus must use protective spectacles. Regular maintenance of apparatus and the possible addition of a silencer can reduce the noise of most laboratory apparatus to acceptable levels. If this is not possible, for example, when noise itself is part of an experiment, attempts should be made to enclose the apparatus in a sealed room or container. The individuals working in this environment should wear earmuffs and work short shifts to reduce exposure. Recommended codes of practice are that exposure when averaged over a 9 hour day should be less than 90 dB. Specific precautions are needed for exposure to a single very large noise, such as gun shots or noise from cartridge-operated tools. Vibration can be a problem with certain chain saws and riveting equipment, this affecting specific fingers with each apparatus. Individuals with known vasospastic disorders should not be allowed to use these tools and careful follow up maintained on workers in these fields.

Heavy apparatus

Lifting apparatus should be available for moving large machinery or the appropriate number of helpers present. Handling of forklift trucks or hoists should be by named personal and they should be parked securely, and the keys locked up when not in use. Fuel, hydraulic, and pneumatic engines require weekly checks, and fibre and metal ropes and chains used for lifting should be checked for fraying, wear, kinks, and twists at least every 6 months. When stacking heavy articles, they should be carefully balanced on secure racks with no protruding ends. Potentially rolling items should be chock-blocked.

Power tools should only be used by personnel who have been trained in these activities and each should know how to stop the apparatus before switching on. Secure guards should be placed over drills, saws, and rotary equipment and these should be checked daily. Workers should not have long loose hair or wear loose clothing, chains, bangles, or uncovered rings.

Where lifting is a regular duty, lifting training should be instituted, together with the use of gloves, solid footwear, and suitable clothing. Loads should be kept as close to the body as possible, lifting with the palms rather than the tips of fingers, and lifting undertaken with the legs, keeping a straight back. The load must not obstruct a person's view and particular care being taken on uneven surfaces, ramps, and stairs.

Gas cylinders are a potential hazard on account of their weight, pressure, and the possible inflammable or toxic properties of their contents. Where heavy cylinders are being used in laboratories suitable holders must be available to avoid rolling or falling; where possible they should be housed outside the laboratory. The gauges must work freely and accurately—it is dangerous to grease any such apparatus. Gas jets must never be directed at a person and cylinders containing dangerous contents should be stored and, where possible, used in a fume chamber. Where air-borne hazardous materials are being used, reference should be made to tables of threshold safety limits.

Structural repairs

Structural work in research areas is usually undertaken by outside contractors who monitor the activities of their employees, particularly in respect to erection of scaffolding, movement across roofs, and avoidance of damage to drains, electric cables, and gas and water pipelines. Many old buildings contain asbestos for lagging, insultating, fireproofing, and cement roof tiles, these require special attention. Nevertheless, the safety officer of an institution has to check fixed ladders for their fixtures and safety loops, the stabilization of free ladders and work platforms, the guard rails of any flat roofs, and the use of harnesses in window cleaning and maintenance work within confined spaces.

Protective clothing

Some form of protective clothing is required in most laboratories. This ranges from the wearing of a laboratory coat to protect personal clothing, to a complete change of clothing and footwear. If there is danger of harmful material touching a worker's skin, rubber or PVC gloves, aprons, goggles, masks, and protective clothing may be worn and suitable screens used. Statutory requirements may exist, for example lead screens may be needed when using X-ray apparatus. Respirators are required with certain dangerous chemicals or bacteria, with complete changes of clothing, showering and passing in and out of the laboratory through an air lock. Appropriate clothing must also be available for all visitors to the laboratory. Care must be taken to secure the valuables of all personnel changing their clothing.

Persons working with toxic chemicals and bacteria or radioactive substances must not eat, drink or smoke in the laboratory and should be warned against pencil chewing, nail biting, label licking, and applying cosmetics. Oral pipetting of such substances must be forbidden and, if a worker's skin or clothing becomes contaminated, thorough washing and decontamination undertaken. Eye-washing kits should be available and visible in these areas. Particular care must be taken when shaking, opening, and pouring out of containers, in order to prevent splashing and contamination of the outside of the container. When an individual is working with any dangerous material a second person should be within hailing distance. Should toxic chemicals, bacteria or radioactive substances come into contact with a person's eyes or skin, the areas should be thoroughly washed with warm water, using soap where appropriated, but taking care not to spread the substance to other areas. Seeking a medical opinion is also advisable.

Operations on infected patients or animals

In the operating room the most likely method of transmission of an infectious disease is by cutting or stabbing of a surgeon or assistant, the so-called needlestick injuries. Particular care must be taken with patients who are known or suspected to have hepatitis B (Australian Antigen), human immunodeficiency virus, or resistant organisms. If personnel are known to be at high risk of exposure to Hepatitis B, immunization should be considered. Similar precautions must be taken when dealing with infected animals, a particular risk being infection with anthrax.

Everyone involved in the procedure must be aware of the potential hazards. All staff must wear disposable aprons, gloves, and overshoes. Scrubbed individuals wear disposable gowns, two pairs of gloves, and a visor. The minimal number of instruments must be used. Extra care should be taken to avoid any stab injuries. Infected blood spilt onto the floor can be detoxicated by the addition of Precept granules. This sodium dichloroisocyanurate product liberates chlorine on contact with water and its powder form turns the blood into a more easily removable gel. The necessary number of bags, bins, and suction-container liners must be available and subsequently all material double bagged and carefully labelled and disposed of as discussed in the following sections. Nondisposable items such as instruments should be washed in running water and then placed in a detergent. Subsequent management is usually by autoclaving but, for materials which withstand autoclaving badly, low pressure steam—and formaldehyde or ethylene oxide sterilization are appropriate. Full cleaning with appropriate detergents should be undertaken of every operating surface and all floors after the procedure. At least 2 hours should be allowed for this cleaning, and time for the detergent to dry and air changes to take place before reusing the area.

Radioactive substances

The use of radioactive substances (radiation sources, radiobiology) is governed by statutory requirements; institutions, personnel, and the materials involved require registration, and radiation protection councillors, advisors, and supervisors must be appointed by the controlling authority. In the UK personnel working with these substances and whose resulting annual dosage might exceed three-tenths of the annual maximum permissible radiation are labelled as classified workers and should attend courses of instruction and be supervised by radiation protection officers. They must be over 16 years of age and be medically and dosimetrically examined, and have their blood and urine tested. Medical examination ensures that they can perform their duties without risk to themselves or others and establishes health status prior to and after commencing such work. Dosimetric examination includes the wearing of film badges (this being a legal requirement) on the chest or waist (under protective clothing where appropriate) and also regular monitoring of skin, hair, and clothes. The dosage exposed to must be assessed by Health and Safety Commission approved laboratories and these recordings accompany the worker to any new place of employment. Maximum permissible doses are stipulated by law and research monitored in the UK by a Centralized National Dose Record Centre.

Safety design is particularly relevant to places handling radioactive material. Employers have a legal requirement to provide suitable and adequate protection to all personnel. It is a legal requirement that radionuclides should only be used in such quantities and in such a form as gives rise to the minimum hazard consistent with the object to be achieved. Transportation distances should be minimal and steps and other obstacles avoided. Movement of sources outside the laboratory area must be strictly under the supervision of staff authorized by employers (in writing) to act for this purpose. Generous space should be allowed and working and floor surfaces smooth. When gaseous radiation substances are in use, fume chambers must be provided and specific ventilation installed. Fire precautions should be worked out with the local fire brigade who should be aware of the local layout and areas of storage. These areas should be well labelled. The working areas, air and instruments, should be frequently monitored for excess activity. Sealed sources are rarely used in animal research. They should be in unbreakable containers and well labelled, and should be carefully recorded and a regular audit of all radioactive material undertaken. Handling of radioactive sources must always be undertaken with the appropriate instruments. Transport of radioactive substances between institutions is legally controlled. Packages must be at least 10 cm square, 'jam proof', shielded, uncontaminated, securely closed and clearly labelled. The number of packages and its total transport index and radiation dose rate are stipulated: to exceed these limits individual permission must be obtained from the Department of the Environment.

Should any spill or leakage occur in the handling of radioactive material it must be fully recorded, all contaminated areas and personnel monitored dosimetrically and medically followed up. Reports should be submitted to the radiation protection advisor. The monitoring and protective measures discussed in this section must also be applied to individuals working with X-rays or radiation beam therapy.

Waste disposal

Planning for the safe disposal of harmful waste must be an integral part of the design of any experimental study. The plan must satisfy the local and national legal requirements, and disposal should be undertaken rapidly once the products have been used or are no longer required. Dangerous waste should be locked up in labelled containers. There should be a periodic review of all hazardous materials stored within the institution as unused material can accumulate, for instance in the back of fume cupboards. Disposal should be undertaken while those persons responsible for any hazardous materials are still in the employment of the institution and while containers are still fully labelled. It is helpful to have an advisor with some chemical knowledge involved in this activity. The involvement of a medical officer or a veterinary surgeon in discussions of prevention and prophylaxis may be appropriate, particularly when dealing with transmissable diseases. An uncommon but inconvenient occurrence is the sensitization of an individual to animal carcasses or protein waste, this should be looked for an avoiding action undertaken before the onset of severe symptoms.

General solid waste

Waste bins should be strategically placed around a laboratory to ensure that they are close to the site of need, yet not interfering with free passage. Sharp instruments such as needles, scalpels, and broken glass must be kept separate from general waste. Many laboratory injuries involve glassware and scalpels. All glassware being disposed of, whether broken or intact, must be placed in a specially provided glass bin. Discarded needles and syringes should be rendered useless to prevent further use, and placed together with disposable blades and other sharp instruments in a sharps box. Glass bins and sharp boxes must be purpose built, well labelled, always available in areas where they are needed, never overfilled and be sealed and disposed of in a prescribed way when they are full. These containers are not reopened and the institution must have arrangements with an appropriate disposing authority. Contaminated instruments must be disposed of in a manner appropriate to the contaminant: combustible substances should be collected separately. Household waste is usually collected and disposed of in black plastic bags and chemical waste in yellow plastic bags: no sharp material or glass should be placed in either type of bag.

General liquid waste: Although the majority of liquid waste products can be discharged into local sewers, certain hazardous materials are unsuitable for this form of disposal. Local authorities should be consulted in cases of doubt. Objectional liquid waste include, large amounts of acids and alkalis (pH below 6 or above 11), substances which have toxic gases, directly or after hydrolysis, substances which are corrosive or toxic by skin absorption, and substantial amounts of water insoluble substances (radioactive materials are considered below). Chlorinated and high oxygen containing solvents and hydrocarbons should be collected separately, since some of these combinations are explosive. All substances requiring alternative methods of disposal should be collected in a well-labelled jar ready for collection by disposal contractors and transported to registered sites. Solid biological waste such as animal carcasses should be disposed of by incineration. If cultures of a microorganism are being handled, it is important to know the biological characteristics and, in appropriate cases, immunization previously undertaken. Any contact with the skin, especially the eyes, nose, or mouth must be avoided. Cultures should be sterilized by disinfection or some other means such as autoclaving, incineration, or filtration. Apparatus must either be cleaned or disposed of, it being dangerous to leave dirty apparatus untreated. All workers have a responsibility to their fellow employees in this respect, some of whom will be less aware of the potential hazards.

Radioactive substances: Disposal of radioactive material is strictly controlled, regulations are related to the nature and quantity of the compounds in use, some flexibility is allowed to suit the local conditions. The carcasses of contaminated animals should be disposed of in an appropriate macerator or incinerator, disposal of this form should be discussed with the local radiation protection officer as, in the UK, there are statutory requirements to keep records of the amount of isotopes disposed of by all the acceptable routes. Compounds with low levels of radiation activity, such as excreta and liquids, can be released in measured quantities directly into the sewers. Similar radiation levels of solid material are allowed into ordinary refuse dumps and gases released into the atmosphere through specific release portals. Higher levels of radioactivity in any form of compound, require collection in labelled suitable jars and arrangements made for removal by special disposal services for storage until, by decay, the activity is reduced to the level which permits discharged in the ordinary way.

Sources of information

The necessity for adequate literature on health and safety at work can not be overemphasized. Complete distribution of the local rules should be statutory and many of the excellent publications on the subject made freely available. These include references 1 and 2 and the additional guidance notes and excellent publications published by Her Majesty's Stationery Office. At a departmental level the safety booklets produced by Imperial College London are very informative and relatively inexpensive. The series covers biological, chemical, electrical, radiation, and workshop hazards. A number of laboratory suppliers provide useful literature. The British Drug Houses produce wall charts with advice on first aid and on how to deal with spillage of hazardous chemicals and the catalogue of the Aldwych Chemical Company contains coded recommendations on disposal of waste quantities and spillage of most chemicals on their list. The above literature and previous statutory details are primarily related to research in the UK. However, the problems are universal and the advice given is appropriate to research carried out worldwide.

Summary

1. In the UK, universities and research institutions are legally required to ensure the health and safety of all staff and visitors in their precinct.
2. Safety is an integral part of research planning and techniques.
3. Reading the published literature on safety will enable the researcher to benefit from previous experience and achieve optimal safety standards.
4. Harmful products should be fully labelled; storage areas should be maintained in the appropriate conditions and the appropriate hazard warning signs displayed.
5. Electrical and heavy appliances should be handled by trained personnel.
6. Operative procedures undertaken on humans or animals infected with transmissable disease require specific techniques to avoid contamination and spread of the disease.
7. Personnel working with radioactive substances require continuous dosimetric monitoring.

8. Harmful substances usually require denaturing by incineration, chemical or isotopic decay before sufficiently low levels can be obtained for discharge with household waste into sewers or into the atmosphere.

References

1. Health and Safety at Work Act (1974). HMSO, London.
2. Committee of Vice Chancellors and Principals (1974). *The Code of practice on safety in universities. HMSO*, London.

Section B:
Data collection and analysis

8. Principles of design and statistics

Overview

Two numerical factors bedevil the biomedical researcher. The first is that measurements of events in the animal kingdom and its environment are subject to wide variation. The second is that the researcher cannot examine complete populations and has to be satisfied with the results obtained from samples. Thus the researcher has to investigate problems by surveys or experiments undertaken on samples taken from wider populations. The theory of statistics is used to assess how reliable sample results reflect what is happening in the population from which they are drawn. The process initially involves placing sample results in an ordered fashion, a process known as descriptive statistics. This is followed by calculating how reliable one can infer that sample results hold for the whole population, a process known as inferential statistics. In order to do this the researcher must understand enough statistics to:

1. plan a survey or experiment and link its design to the proposed analysis;
2. undertake descriptive analysis and present the data in an easily recordable and understandable way, using both pictorial (graphical) and tabular methods;
3. comprehend the principles of inferential statistics;
4. apply the appropriate statistical tests;
5. discuss problems with a statistician, using unambiguous language and making sure that the right problem(s) is (are) being examined;
6. understand and criticize statistical reports at meetings and in the literature.

The application of statistics does not necessarily require a sophisticated understanding of mathematics, rather it requires: sound logic, together with a keen eye for unexpected trends in data; an understanding of statistical concepts; the ability to make use of a limited number of algebraic formulae, and the ability to carry out computations. The last of these requirements is usually undertaken with the use of a calculator or computer, especially when there are large amounts of data.

Principles of investigation

In Section A research was defined as asking questions and investigating possible answers. Three types of questions are generally asked:

1. What produces an effect?
2. What is the size of the effect?
3. What produces the best effect?

The subject of 'what' and the 'effect' are termed variables. The 'what' variable is known as the *independent variable* (also sometimes referred to as the explanatory or predictor variable) and the 'effect' variable as the *dependent variable* (also sometimes known as the response or outcome variable). To answer Question 1 the researcher examines whether a change in a dependent variable is associated with a given change in an independent variable or group of variables. To answer Question 2 the researcher has to measure the size of this change. However to answer Question 3 the researcher has to compare the sizes of the various changes in a dependent variable, or group of variables associated with various changes in different independent variables or groups of variables.

Figure 8.1 shows an example of how changes in a dependent variable can be associated with changes in an independent variable (Question 1). The line is known as a regression line from which the expected amount of change in the dependent variable can be calculated for given changes in the independent variable (Question 2). The scatter about the line gives an indication of the variability of these expected changes. Question 3 is answered by examining the effect on the dependent variable of more than one independent variable. Sometimes a no treatment group is included to act as a *control group*; this control group then provides a baseline against which to judge the effect of any change in the independent variable.

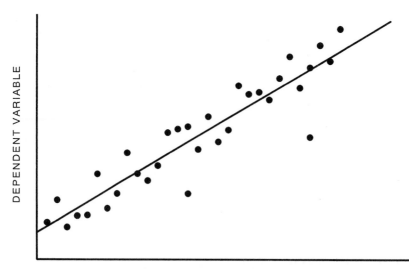

INDEPENDENT VARIABLE

Fig. 8.1 Association of variables—scatter diagram.

Principles of design

Investigations may be carried out in one of two ways: (a) by means of a survey or (b) by means of a controlled experiment.

(a) By means of a *survey*: this involves collecting evidence from naturally occurring events, which are taking, or have already taken place. The application of a survey to the three research questions is demonstrated in the following KPH examples (see p. 5):

Question 1 What produces an effect?

In this case the feeding of KPH to the puppy is the 'what' or independent variable and the energy level of the puppy is the dependent variable. By carrying out a survey among puppy owners who feed their puppies KPH it may be possible to establish whether changes in the amount of KPH are associated with different energy levels. However, this method is not very satisfactory unless strict control is kept on how the respondents were chosen and that a correct balance is kept on the different type of puppy being fed KPH, for example the change in energy level produced by a given amount of KPH could well be different for different breeds of puppy or within the same breed at different ages.

Question 2 What is the size of the effect?

Here the actual change in energy level produced by a given change in level of KPH would need to be measured.

Question 3 What produces the best effect?

Here the various types of food product are the independent variables and the puppies preference is the dependent variable. A survey among all puppy owners could possibly establish which food product is the most preferred but again extreme caution must be taken, as not all puppies would have been tested on all the products and some owners could be prejudiced by advertising, maker's name, or even things like the shape and colour of the pack. What a survey of this type will tell one, is what animal foods are being used to feed puppies and the amount used, i.e. it indicates owners' preference, brand share, and consumer habits. It will not indicate which is the 'best' animal food, because of all the extraneous factors (prejudices) which go to make up choice of animal food. (Note: results of surveys can be most misleading as the data derived from them is subject to unknown biases. They can, however, often be extremely useful in suggesting hypotheses for further testing.)

(b) By means of a controlled *experiment*: this involves controlling one or more independent variables and measuring the effects. If experiments are used to cover the three types of question in the KPH study the questions can then be answered in the following way:

Question 1 'What' (KPH = independent variable) produces 'an effect' (energy level = dependent variable). Here the amount of KPH being fed to each breed and age of puppy is precisely controlled, with no extraneous feeding, and an association is looked for between the feeding of KPH and the puppy's energy.

Question 2 The changes in energy level for different levels of KPH can then be measured.

Question 3 'What' (food product: KPH or alternative = independent variables) produces the 'best effect' (puppy's preference = dependent variable). In this case a balanced random set of puppies are allowed a free choice of two or more food products and their preferences studied.

It will be noted that the same examples have been used for both surveys and experiments, however, the differences are very important. In surveys, the information is collected from naturally occurring events, the researcher having *no control* over the amount or type of food product presented to the puppy, and no knowledge of whether the effect is really due, for example, to the neighbour's cat food. In the designed experiment, the food is delivered in a *controlled fashion* and it is possible to eliminate extraneous factors which could bias the result, i.e. *experiments control the 'what' of the question being studied* and randomize (i.e. free from bias) any other extraneous influences. In other words, the results of well-designed randomized experiments are automatically valid as being free from bias and, providing the sample was drawn at random, they can generally be applied to the population from which the sample was drawn. On the other hand the results of a survey would need validation from outside sources to ensure that they are applicable to a wider population than just the sample studied in the survey. (Note: the above examples are given for illustrative purposes only and have not been designed or controlled as rigorously as they would have been in practice.)

Surveys may be undertaken on retrospective or prospective information, whereas experiments are always prospective. The planned prospective experiment also allows precise measurement of the effect to a degree that is hardly ever possible in surveys. Moreover, properly designed experiments will enable one to measure or eliminate interactions between the independent variables, i.e. establish whether the effect of independent variable X is changed in any way by the giving of independent variable Y, and vice versa. (Note: the word control is thus used in research in two ways: to reduce or eliminate outside influence on variables and to denote a control group for comparison.) The main function of a survey is, as its name implies, to survey a population to establish what is currently happening in that population. The main function of a controlled experiment is to try and establish relationships between variables.

Why statistics?

In discussing the principles of investigation no direct mention has so far been made of the science of statistics. However, an implicit assumption has been made, i.e. that it is possible to survey or carry out an experiment on *all* members of a *population*; where, a population is defined as all objects, subjects, or events with specific characteristics, i.e. a statistical population is not necessarily confined to an animal or human population. However, although maximum information would be available if a survey or an experiment was undertaken on all members of the population, this is very seldom possible, as a statistical population can be hypothetical, theoretical, too big or unavailable. Often it would be too costly to test or examine every member, and in some cases, members of the population might be adversely affected by an experiment, making it undesirable to undertake such a study. Hence the need to do research on *samples*, taken from the population under review and to infer from the results of these samples certain characteristics of the population. The problems of inference from samples are further compounded by the great variation in all biological measurements from animals and their environment. Thus, to make a prediction about a population based on the fragmentary evidence of a sample, the sampling has to be carried out with great care and follow certain principles—these principles are part of the science of statistics.

The use of samples gives rise to three main problems:

(a) how to ensure the validity of a sample, i.e. that it is truly *representative* of the population from which it is drawn so that the results taken from the sample can be applied to the population as a whole;

(b) how to assess the *reliability* of the sample results, i.e. how similar would the result be from other samples drawn from the same population;

(c) how to assess whether the effects found between or within samples actually exist or not in the population from which the samples are drawn.

Statistical theory attempts to overcome these problems by using two inter-related techniques. These are known respectively as *descriptive* and *inferential* statistics. These techniques enable the researcher to:

(a) be reasonably sure that a sample is likely to be representative of the population from which it is drawn;

(b) quantify the errors involved in generalizing from a sample to a population;

(c) decide whether to accept or reject any given hypothesis.

Summary

1. In research three types of question are usually asked:
   (a) What produces an effect?
   (b) What is the size of the effect?
   (c) What produces the best effect?

2. The subject of 'what' and the 'effect' are termed variables. The 'what' variable is known as the independent variable and the 'effect' variable is known as the dependent variable.

3. Investigations may be carried out in one of two ways: surveys or controlled experiments.

4. Both surveys and experiments are concerned with assessing the characteristics of a population and how specific factors influence them.

5. Surveys are mainly used to assess what is happening in a given population. Controlled experiments are used to assess what changes are associated with given extraneous factors (independent variables).

6. The researcher is normally looking for what changes take place in a dependent variable arising from a change in an independent variable(s).

7. Investigations of the effects are undertaken on samples chosen from a given population and statistical techniques are used to (a) make reasonably sure that the samples are likely to be valid, i.e. representative of the population from which they have been drawn, (b) determine what would happen in the population, based on the results obtained from these samples and, (c) accept or reject any given hypothesis about the population.

8. A statistical population is not necessarily a human population but is a collective term for all objects, subjects or events with one or more specified characteristics.

9. Statistics can be considered under two inter-related subdivisions: (a) descriptive and (b) inferential (see Chapters 9 and 10).

9. Descriptive statistics

Overview

The function of descriptive statistics is to make sense of a mass of data about the problem at hand. Its role is to present sample data in a convenient, usable and understandable form; in other words to *communicate its meaning* to the researcher as well as to other scientists. Noticing unexpected trends in the sample data and finding out their cause can lead to important new discoveries. This chapter is concerned with some of the commonly used and most useful techniques of descriptive statistics. The first step in the process is to order and group a set of sample measurements, so that their shape, spread and symmetry can be assessed: the shape formed is known as the *sample distribution*. This must not be confused with a sampling distribution which is described in more detail in Chapter 10 (on inferential statistics) and is principally used for making inferences from samples. A common shape for a sample distribution in biological science is a *bell-shaped distribution* where the highest proportion of measurements is in the middle and the smallest proportions are at either end. In many cases this type of distribution can be approximated by the *normal distribution* whose characteristics are described in more detail on p. 88. Sample distributions can be summarized by measures known as statistics of which the more generally used are (a) measures of *central tendency*, such as mean, mode, and median, and (b) measures of *dispersion* such as the standard deviation. Moreover by using standardized measurements (p. 80) distributions using different measurement scales can be compared. When a distribution is converted into standard measurements, a *standard distribution* is said to be obtained. This always has a mean of 0 and a standard deviation of 1. This distribution has fixed proportions between any given standard measurements, and this fact is used in the application and the interpretation of a number of statistical tests.

Determining the shape and pattern of data

The diastolic blood pressure readings in Fig. 9.1 were recorded in a sample of 60 hypertensive patients. Measurements were taken to the nearest 5 mm/Hg. In order to make some visual sense of this data, it is necessary to arrange them in the systematic fashion shown in Fig. 9.2. All the values are listed, usually lowest to highest and a tally mark is placed alongside the measurement every time it occurs (where there are more than five individual measurements these are grouped in fives thus ⅡⅡⅡ). It should be noted that whenever a frequency table is constructed it should always have a title and the units or measurements must always be stated and

Fig. 9.1 Diastolic Blood Pressure Readings* taken from 60 Hypertensive Patients

165, 130, 125, 140, 130, 115, 145, 130, 120, 130
105, 130, 130, 135, 145, 120, 125, 135, 125, 125
120, 140, 155, 135, 110, 140, 115, 115, 135, 120
100, 155, 120, 130, 115, 130, 130, 125, 130, 125
150, 145, 130, 120, 125, 130, 140, 135, 125, 130
135, 130, 140, 140, 135, 150, 150, 145, 130, 110

* to nearest 5 mm/Hg

Fig. 9.2 Frequency Table of Diastolic Blood Pressure of 60 Hypertensive Patients units to nearest 5 mm/Hg

x	Tally	Frequency (f)
100	1	1
105	1	1
110	11	2
115	1111	4
120	1111 1	6
125	1111 111	8
130	1111 1111 1111	15
135	1111 11	7
140	1111 1	6
145	1111	4
150	111	3
155	11	2
160		0
165	1	1
Total = n		60

Where
x represents the different values of the variable. In this case diastolic blood pressure measured in mm/Hg.
(f) is the frequency of occurrence of each of the values of the variable. n is the total number of measurements. In this case 60.

quoted when a value of the variable is given. Note also that if tally marks are made in the way shown above they provide pictorial representation of the sample or frequency distribution one is studying. It is also important to note that the value of a continuous variable (x), given in a table, is the midpoint of a range. In the above example as measurements were taken to the nearest 5 mm/Hg, each value is actually $x \pm 2.5$ mm/Hg so that for example $x = 135$ is actually $132.5 < x \leqslant 137.5$ mm/Hg or $132.5 \leqslant x < 137.5$ mm/Hg, depending on the rule selected for rounding. For the purpose of the example we shall take the range as $132.5 < x \leqslant 137.5$ mm/Hg.

Figure 9.2 has been constructed from the original data and has 14 values of *x*. In cases involving a large number of measurements, the number of values of *x* can also be large and unmanageable. In these cases the *x*'s have to be grouped together into wider bands called 'class intervals'. The resultant table is known as a *grouped frequency table* and each *x* is then taken as the midpoint of the wider class interval. (Note: it is advisable to make all class intervals the same width as this adds considerably to visual understanding. Care must also be taken when drawing conclusions from grouped data, as different groupings can sometimes give different visual effects.)

In general an odd number of class intervals should be chosen with the midpoint of the centre interval as near as possible to the arithmetic mean of the distribution. The arithmetic mean ($\bar{x}$) of a distribution is obtained by summing all the measurements and dividing by the total number of measurements, i.e.

$$\bar{x} = \sum_{i}^{n} \frac{x_i}{n}$$

or if calculated from a frequency table:

$$\bar{x} = \sum_{i}^{n} \frac{(f_i x_i)}{n}$$

where f_i is the frequency in the *i*th group or cell. In the example given, $\bar{x} =$ 130.75 mm/Hg. Figures 9.3–9.5 are examples of grouped frequency distributions taken from the sample of 60 measurements shown in Fig. 9.2. Note how in Fig. 9.4 (b) and 9.5 (b), where the central value is near the mean of the distribution, a much more symmetrical distribution is obtained.

Fig.9.3 Diastolic Blood Pressure Grouped in Intervals of 10 mm/Hg

Class Width	*x*	*f*
97.5< – ≤ 107.5	102.5	2
107.5< – ≤ 117.5	112.5	6
117.5< – ≤ 127.5	122.5	14
127.5< – ≤ 137.5	132.5	22
137.5< – ≤ 147.5	142.5	10
147.5< – ≤ 157.5	152.5	5
157.5< – ≤ 167.5	162.5	1
	n	60

The first column 'Class Width' is shown for illustration, it is not usually given.

Fig. 9.4 Diastolic Blood Pressure Grouped in Intervals of 15 mm/Hg

(a) Starting at 100 mm/Hg		(b) Starting at 95 mm/Hg	
x	f	x	f
105	4	100	2
120	18	115	12
135	28	130	30
150	9	145	13
165	1	160	3
n	60	n	60

Fig. 9.5 Diastolic Blood Pressure Grouped in Intervals of 25 mm/Hg

(a) Starting at 100 mm/Hg		(b) Starting at 95 mm/Hg	
x	f	x	f
110	14	105	8
135	40	130	42
160	6	155	10
n	60	n	60

Graphing techniques

Having constructed a frequency distribution from a set of raw data, it is helpful to present the distribution in pictorial form so that its essential features can be more readily seen. Figure 9.6 shows a *histogram* for the blood-pressure data, and Fig. 9.7 the same data displayed in the form of a *frequency polygon*. In the latter, a dot is placed where the top of the middle of the bar of the histogram would have been. For a histogram, frequency is represented by the area of a bar, or the height, if the widths of bars are equal and are considered as one unit each. In frequency polygons, frequency is represented by the area under the curve between two points on the curve. It is important to remember this fact, as it is used later in this chapter. When two or more frequency distributions are compared, the frequency polygon usually provides a clearer picture of their shape but a histogram gives a better comparison of class frequencies.

To avoid misrepresentation and over or under emphasis of particular differences in any pictorial representation, a baseline must always be shown and all comparisons should be on a linear basis, for example height with width constant but not area or volume, as the latter are very difficult to judge visually. For the same reason, the three-quarter high rule is often used for graphic representation of a fre-

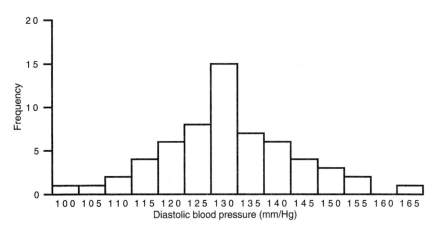

Fig. 9.6 Histogram.

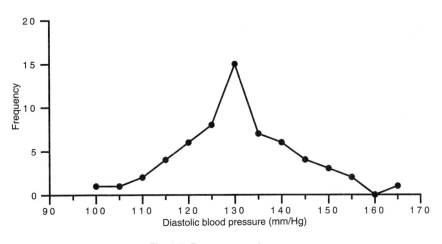

Fig. 9.7 Frequency polygon.

quency distribution. This means that in plotting the frequencies, the vertical axis should be laid out so that the height of the maximum point (representing the measurement or category with the highest frequency) is approximately equal to three-quarters the length of the horizontal axis.

The blood pressure measurements used in the previous example come from a continuous variable, i.e. one with no natural breaks. If the variable being measured is discrete, i.e. noncontinuous or if an *ordinal scale,* such as a rating scale, is considered, a *bar graph* should be drawn rather than a histogram and the bars should be separated, so as to avoid the implications of continuity among the categories. For the same reason, it is inappropriate to draw a frequency polygon to represent ordinal data. As before, the area of each bar is used to represent the frequency for that category. By way of illustration, suppose that the 60 patients with hypertension were administered a new drug to see if it reduces their blood pressure. As one indicator of side effects, the patients could be asked to rate how they feel on a four-point scale, where four represents the most negative feeling, one the most positive, and three and two are somewhere in between. The frequency responses could have been as follows:

x	f
1	21
2	15
3	18
4	6
n	60

These findings are represented pictorially by the bar chart in Fig. 9.8 and indicate that only 10 per cent of patients suffered negative side effects but 35 per cent achieved a very positive feeling.

If the frequency distribution is a *nominally scaled* variable (i.e. where the scaling is done using a variable in which there is no set order, for example by colours), the various categories can be represented along the horizontal axis in any order, but care must be taken not to arrange the data in an order which purports to show relationships which are not there. Frequency distributions take on many different shapes. In the biological sciences, measurements of a variable, such as blood pres-

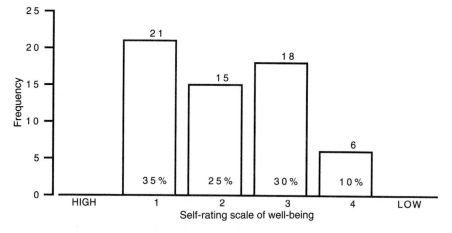

Fig. 9.8 Bar chart of responses of patients to feeling of well-being after the administration of a new drug.

sure, more often than not result in a bell-shaped frequency distribution, like that shown in Fig. 9.9. Such a bell-shaped curve is by definition symmetrical (i.e. if folded in half along the vertical axis, the two sides coincide) with the majority of readings of the variable occurring in the middle of the range (as with the blood pressure illustration). When a distribution is not symmetrical (Fig. 9.10), it is said to be *skewed*. If the distribution tails off at the high end of the horizontal axis, in other words there are relatively few frequencies at this end, it is said to be positively skewed. A negatively skewed distribution has few frequencies at the low end of the horizontal axis.

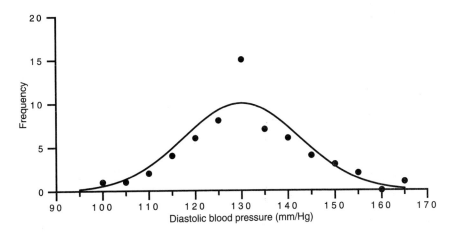

Fig. 9.9 Normal distribution curve fitted to the blood pressure measurements from Fig. 9.2.

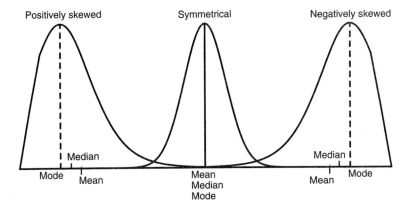

Fig. 9.10 Skewed distributions.

Summary statistics of frequency distributions

So far the analytical methods used have been simply to organize data into a meaningful and useful form by tabulation and graphing. This gives each individual measurement some meaning, in that it provides a 'picture' of how similar or different it is from the rest of the measurements in the sample. This is not, however, usually sufficient and a method needs to be found of describing a distribution by way of its important characteristics. Most frequency distributions can be meaningfully summarized by some measure of *central tendency* and some measure of *dispersion* around the selected measure of central tendency.

Measures of central tendency

There are three main measures of central tendency

1. the mode
2. the median
3. the arithmetic mean.

1. the mode (mo)

The mode is the value of the variable which occurs with greatest frequency. In discrete variables the mode is always an exact figure, but in continuous variables it has to be calculated and, depending on the degree of accuracy needed the method of calculation varies. The great advantage of the mode is that a rough value can be arrived at fairly easily by inspection. It is, therefore, a useful first indicator of central tendency when running an eye over a sample of data to quickly get some feel for it. Its disadvantage is that its value is often based on only one value of the variable, albeit the most frequently occurring one, and therefore full use is not being made of all the data. It is moreover not easily amenable to mathematical analysis or manipulation, and hence its use in hypothesis testing is fairly limited. For the sample of 60 patients with hypertension (Fig. 9.2) shows the frequency with which each measurement occurred. From it, it can easily be seen that the modal value is 130 mm/Hg. A more precise value can be calculated taking into account the values on either side of the mode. This calculation gives the modal value as 129.8 mm/Hg.

2. The median (med)

The median (med) is another indicator of central tendency. It is the midpoint measurement of the distribution, i.e. it is the value of the variable above and below which one-half of the frequencies fall. For the sample of 60 patients with hypertension, when all the measurements are arranged in order: the median lies between the 30th and 31st measurement counting from either the top or the bottom. The value of the median is obtained by producing a cumulative frequency table as in Fig. 9.11

Fig. 9.11 Cumulative Fequency Table of Diastolic
Blood Pressure units to nearest 5 mm/Hg

x	f	165 Σf 100	100 Σf 165
100	1	1	60
105	1	2	59
110	2	4	58
115	4	8	56
120	6	14	52
125	8	22	46
130	15	37	38
135	7	44	23
140	6	50	16
145	4	54	10
150	3	57	6
155	2	59	3
160	0	59	1
165	1	60	1

from which it can be seen that the median for 60 patients with hypertension is 130 mm/Hg. If there had been an odd number of measurements, the median would have been found by taking the value corresponding to the middle measurement; for example had there been 61 measurements the median would have been the value of the variable corresponding to the 31st measurement. Calculations from grouped data often give a slightly different and less accurate result than using ungrouped data, because of the estimation involved: but it is a much faster method of calculation when a very large sample is used. Like the mode, it is inelegant mathematically, and is not dependent on the values of the variable, thus like the mode it is little used in significance or hypothesis testing. Its main use is when describing highly skewed distributions, such as income distributions, when extreme values make nonsense of any arithmetic mean (see below). For continuous variables a more accurate way of calculating the median, taking into account its position within the class interval, is available. This method gives the median value of the 60 patients with hypertension as 130.17 mm/Hg.

3. The arithmetic mean ($\bar{x}$)

The most commonly used measure of central tendency is the arithmetic mean or average. It is the most useful measure, because it uses all the values of a measurement within a sample and is highly amenable to mathematical analysis. Its behaviour in sampling can be mathematically established, thus making it ideal for significance and hypothesis testing. The mean is the sum of the sample values of a measure, divided by the number in the sample. For the sample of 60 measures of diastolic blood pressure:

$$\bar{x} = \frac{100 + 105 + (2 \times 110) + (4 \times 115) + \ldots 165}{60}$$

$$= 130.75 \ (0) \ \text{mm/Hg}$$

$\bar{x}$ (referred to as x bar) is the usual notation for the arithmetic mean. It should be noted that when carrying out statistical procedures, all intermediary calculations should be done using one decimal place more than is required in the final answer. (Since, at a later step the mean of the diastolic blood pressure sample will be used as part of another calculation, the third place of decimal is given here in brackets.) When not using a calculator or computer it is faster to calculate the arithmetic mean from grouped data than ungrouped data, but the method is less accurate as it involves some degree of estimation as the midpoints of the class intervals are taken as the values of x. The arithmetic mean is the value of the variable which balances all the values of the measurements on either side of it, i.e. it is the centre of gravity. In this sense it is analogous to the pivot of a seesaw. Note, a really extreme value of a measurement to one side of it, can change the value of the mean (the position of the pivot) very markedly so that although the mean is the most used measure of central tendency in statistics, the median is often preferred when the distribution is very skewed, since it is much less sensitive to extreme values.

When a distribution is a symmetrical bell-shaped distribution, the mean, median, and mode all take the same value. In the example of the 60 patients with hypertension, the mean diastolic blood pressure is 130.75 mm/Hg, the median diastolic blood pressure is 130.17 mm/Hg, and the modal diastolic blood pressure 129.8 mm/Hg. This suggests that the data is slightly skewed. Since the mean is higher than the median, which in turn is higher than the mode, the skew is a positive one.

The degree of dispersion of a set of data

Measures of central tendency are calculated in order to obtain one value which will typify a distribution. The more compact the individual readings around the measure of central tendency the more this measure typifies the data. Comparing an individual measurement against the measure of central tendency provides evidence as to how similar this individual measurement is to the others in the sample. The more compact the data, the less extreme an individual measurement is from the mean before it is considered to be exceptional: this is shown in Fig. 9.12.

Measures of dispersion

Measures of *dispersion* provide a way of expressing quantatively how compact or otherwise is a set of data.

1. *The range.* One such measure of dispersion is the range, this is the difference between the largest and smallest measurement. In the sample of diastolic blood

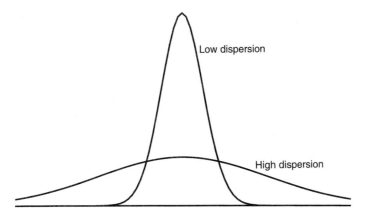

Fig. 9.12 Degrees of dispersion.

pressures the highest blood pressure is 165 mm/Hg and the lowest is 100 mm/Hg. The range is therefore 165–100 mm/Hg or 65 mm/Hg. The chief advantage of the range is that it is easily and quickly found, and is therefore a good measure to use when initially getting the feel of some new data. Its main disadvantage as a measure of dispersion is its instability. One extreme measurement in a sample will result in a large range, even though the rest of the measurements are very compact. In repeated sampling, the arithmetic mean of the range of a set of samples of the same size is known as the mean range, it can be useful as an estimator of the population standard deviation.

2. *Mean deviation (MD)*. Another approach to measuring dispersion, making use of all the values of a measurement within a sample, is to take the sum of each value's deviation from the mean, irrespective of sign, and to divide this total by the number of values in the sample, i.e. $\Sigma |x - \bar{x}| / n$. This provides the average or mean deviation from the mean. Note that deviations have to be taken irrespective of sign, otherwise, by definition of the mean, the sum would be 0. This measure is very rarely used as it is not very amenable to mathematical manifestation.

3. *Standard deviation (SD)*. A far more practical way of eliminating the negative signs is to square the differences so that:

$$\Sigma \frac{f|x - \bar{x}|}{n} \text{ becomes } \Sigma \frac{f(x - \bar{x})^2}{n}$$

This measure is known as the variance (σ^2 or var) of the distribution. The square root of the variance is known as the standard deviation (SD) and is the measure overwhelmingly used to describe the dispersion of a distribution about its mean:

$$SD = \left[\Sigma \frac{f(x - \bar{x})^2}{n} \right]^{\frac{1}{2}}$$

A more exact method for estimating the population variance and standard deviation from a sample, is to divide the sample sum of squares by $(n-1)$ rather than n, and the $(n-1)$ division should always be used when calculations are made from samples. In the example of diastolic blood pressure, the best estimate of the population variance is 158.3263 mm/Hg and the standard deviation is 12.583 mm/Hg.

Standardization

Mention has already been made of the standard deviation being the companion measure to the arithmetic mean. If the mean diastolic blood pressure is 135.70 mm/Hg, a reading of 145 mm/Hg is 14.25 mm/Hg above the mean. How extreme a value this is depends on how dispersed are the readings around the central tendency. In the example of the 60 diastolic blood pressures, the calculated value for the standard deviation is 12.583 mm/Hg. This means that the reading of 145 mm/Hg is 14.25/12.583 standard deviation units above the mean, or 1.132 standard units above the mean. The process of dividing the deviation of a score from its mean by the standard deviation, is known as standardizing or transforming to z scores or standard scores. The great advantage of standard scores is that they represent deviations from the mean in standard units, instead of the original units in which the measurements were taken. This conversion enables the position of a subject on one variable to be compared with its position on a second variable, even though the units of measurement for the two variables are different. Two important properties of the distribution of standard scores are that its mean is always zero and its standard deviation always equals one.

The standard normal distribution

Because of the importance of the normal distribution the proportions of a variable lying between the mean and any standard score have been calculated and tabulated (Fig. 9.13), so that by converting measures of a normally distributed variable to standard scores, the effective proportion of values lying between the mean and any value can be calculated. This is because in a standard normal distribution the total area under the curve is equal to 1 and the proportion between any two given standard scores is constant. Thus a fixed proportion of readings always lie under the curve between the mean and a given point above or below the mean.
In particular:

1. Between the mean and one standard deviation above or one standard deviation below the mean, are found 34.13 per cent of all measurements. In other words 68.26 per cent of all measurements lie between −1.00 and +1.00 standard deviations from the mean.

2. Between the mean and two standard deviations above or two standard deviations below the mean, lie 47.725 per cent of all measurements. So, 95.45 per cent of all measurements occur between −2.00 and +2.00 standard deviations from the mean. (Note 95 per cent of all measurements lie between $\bar{x} \pm 1.96$ SD.)

Fig. 9.13 Table of the area under the normal curve

$\dfrac{x}{\sigma}$	0.00	0.01	0.02	0.03	0.04	0.05	0.06	0.07	0.08	0.09
0.0	.000	.0040	.0080	.0120	.0159	.0199	.0239	.0279	.0319	.0359
0.1	.0398	.0438	.0478	.0517	.0557	.0596	.0636	.0675	.0714	.0753
0.2	.0793	.0832	.0871	.0910	.0948	.0987	.1026	.1064	.1103	.1141
0.3	.1179	.1217	.1255	.1293	.1331	.1368	.1406	.1443	.1480	.1517
0.4	.1554	.1591	.1628	.1664	.1700	.1736	.1772	.1808	.1844	.1879
0.5	.1915	.1950	.1985	.2019	.2054	.2088	.2133	.2157	.2190	.2224
0.6	.2257	.2291	.2324	.2357	.2389	.2422	.2454	.2486	.2518	.2549
0.7	.2580	.2611	.2642	.2673	.2704	.2734	.2764	.2794	.2823	.2852
0.8	.2881	.2910	.2939	.2967	.2995	.3023	.3051	.3078	.3106	.3133
0.9	.3159	.3186	.3212	.3238	.3264	.3289	.3315	.3340	.3365	.3389
1.0	.3413	.3438	.3461	.3485	.3508	.3531	.3554	.3577	.3599	.3621
1.1	.3643	.3665	.3686	.3708	.3729	.3749	.3770	.3790	.3810	.3830
1.2	.3849	.3869	.3888	.3907	.3925	.3944	.3962	.3980	.3997	.4015
1.3	.4032	.4049	.4066	.4082	.4099	.4115	.4131	.4147	.4162	.4177
1.4	.4192	.4207	.4222	.4236	.4251	.4265	.4279	.4292	.4306	.4319
1.5	.4332	.4345	.4357	.4370	.4382	.4394	.4406	.4418	.4430	.4441
1.6	.4452	.4463	.4474	.4485	.4495	.4505	.4515	.4525	.4535	.4545
1.7	.4554	.4564	.4573	.4582	.4591	.4599	.4608	.4616	.4625	.4633
1.8	.4641	.4649	.4656	.4664	.4671	.4678	.4686	.4693	.4699	.4706
1.9	.4713	.4719	.4726	.4732	.4738	.4744	.4750	.4756	.4762	.4767
2.0	.4772	.4778	.4783	.4788	.4793	.4798	.4803	.4808	.4812	.4817
2.1	.4821	.4826	.4830	.4834	.4838	.4842	.4846	.4850	.4854	.4857
2.2	.4861	.4865	.4868	.4871	.4875	.4878	.4881	.4884	.4887	.4890
2.3	.4893	.4896	.4898	.4901	.4904	.4906	.4909	.4911	.4913	.4916
2.4	.4918	.4920	.4922	.4925	.4927	.4929	.4931	.4932	.4934	.4936
2.5	.4938	.4940	.4941	.4943	.4945	.4946	.4948	.4949	.4951	.4952
2.6	.4953	.4955	.4956	.4957	.4959	.4960	.4961	.4962	.4963	.4964
2.7	.4965	.4966	.4967	.4968	.4969	.4970	.4971	.4972	.4973	.4974
2.8	.4974	.4975	.4976	.4977	.4977	.4978	.4979	.4980	.4980	.4981
2.9	.4981	.4982	.4983	.4983	.4984	.4984	.4985	.4985	.4986	.4986
3.0	.49865	.4987	.4987	.4988	.4988	.4989	.4989	.4989	.4990	.4990
3.1	.49903	.4991	.4991	.4991	.4992	.4992	.4992	.4992	.4993	.4993

3. Between the mean and three standard deviations above or three standard deviations below the mean, are found 49.865 per cent of all measurements. So, 99.73 per cent of all measurements lie between −3.00 and +3.00 standard deviations from the mean. (Note 99.8 per cent of all observations lie between $\bar{x} \pm 3.075$SD).

By using a standardized normal distribution (Curve) (Fig. 9.13), it is possible to determine the percentage of measurements between any two standard scores. Taking the reading of diastolic blood pressure of 145 mm/Hg, which was found to be 1.132 standard units above the mean, and using the normal curve table: between the mean and +1.132 standard deviations lies 0.3708 proportion of all measurements in the distribution, or 37.08 per cent. The importance of these findings in assessing the significance of any reading will be described in more detail in the chapters on inferential statistics and statistical testing. It is essential to note that transforming initial measurements to standard scores does not in any way change the form of the original distribution. All it does is to convert the mean to zero and the standard deviation to one. Thus, if the original distribution of measurements is not normal, the distribution of standard scores will also not be normal. Use can be made of this to determine whether a set of data really does form a normal distribution, i.e. one can undertake a 'goodness of fit' test to examine whether the data conforms to a given hypothetical distribution (p. 103). The fact that a set of data does form a normal distribution is an important finding, since in using many of the powerful parametric inferential techniques discussed in the chapter on inferential statistics, one of the conditions to be satisfied is that measurements are drawn from normally distributed populations.

Summary

1. A frequency distribution gives an immediate overview of the shape of a set of measurements.

2. Interval data can be presented visually using histograms or frequency polygons. Ordinal data, such as rating scales, is best presented as a bar graph arranged in ascending order of the rating scale. Nominal data can also be presented visually by bar graphs, the various categories being in any order provided it is not biased.

3. Three measures of central tendency are the mode, median, and arithmetic mean. The mode is the value of the variable occurring with greatest frequency. The median is the value of the variable above and below which half of the measurements fall. The arithmetic mean is the centre of gravity of the distribution, i.e. it is the value of the variable which balances all the measurements on either side of it (in this sense being analogous to the pivot of a seesaw): it is, however sensitive to extreme values of measurement. Except when there are extreme values of a measurement at one end of a distribution, giving the distribution a very positive or negative skew, the mean is the most used measure of central tendency. For a symmetrical bell-shaped distribution the mean, median, and mode all take the same value.

4. Three measures of dispersion are the range, the mean deviation, and the standard deviation: the standard deviation is by far the most useful measure.

5. A standard score measures the distance of an individual measurement from its mean in terms of its standard deviation. This process is known as standardization and all distribution that have been standardized have:
    (a) an area under the curve equal to 1;
    (b) a mean of 0 and a SD of 1
    (c) a fixed proportion of measurements between any two points on the horizon-

tal axis.

6. The standard normal curve, apart from the properties noted above, has the following important properties:

(a) it is symmetrical;

(b) its arithmetic mean, median, and mode are equal;

(c) the proportions lying between its mean and any other point have been extensively calculated and published. In particular:

— 68.26 per cent of all measurements lie between −1.00 and +1.00 standard deviations from the mean.

— 95.45 per cent of all measurements lie between −2.00 and +2.00 standard deviations from the mean (95 per cent between ± 1.96 SD).

— 99.73 per cent of all measurements lie between −3.00 and +3.00 standard deviations from the mean (99.8 per cent between ± 3.075 SD).

Use can be made of these properties to test whether (a) a sample of measurements really does form a normal distribution and (b) whether any particular measurement is more likely or less likely to have come from a particular distribution.

10. Inferential statistics

Overview

In the last chapter, by using descriptive statistics, a mass of data was analysed and digested so that its main characteristics could be easily grasped and understood. In this chapter these ideas are developed to show how, by the use of what are known as inferential statistics, statements can be made, with varying degrees of confidence, about the parent population from which the data is drawn. By doing so, it is possible to assess the probability as to whether any hypothesis being tested should be accepted or rejected, or whether or not any new data that comes to hand can be regarded as coming from the same population. The ability to make inferential statements from a sample is based on the fact that the *sampling distributions* of the descriptive statistics of any sample can be derived theoretically and that these sampling distributions have not only been derived but have also been extensively tabulated. This means that the expected variation and probability of occurrence of any statistic on repeated sampling is known and tabulated, so that by reference to the appropriate table it is possible to estimate whether any particular sample or value from a sample is representative of the population from which it is thought to have been drawn. To put it another way round, it is possible to infer from a sample, the populations from which it could have come, or the populations from which it is unlikely to have come. Thus it is possible to determine on the one hand the probability of a sample coming from any given population and, on the other, to draw confidence limits or intervals around a sample, and infer that the sample would be most unlikely to have come from a population whose parameters lie outside these limits.

Sampling distributions

Sampling distributions are theoretical distributions mainly used for drawing inferences from samples and must not be confused with sample distributions as defined in Chapter 9. The latter are empirical distributions and are mainly used for descriptive and illustrative purposes. Research is usually undertaken on samples and the resulting sample statistics are used to estimate population parameters. This procedure is known as statistical inference. If a series of samples are taken at random from a given population, the frequency distribution of each sample will vary and, even though most samples will have characteristics very similar to those of the parent population, a few will be markedly different. In some cases marked differences would have occurred by chance but, it is not unreasonable to suppose that in other cases samples with different characteristics have come from a different parent population or populations. Statistical inference enables one to assess the probabilities as to whether differences have occurred by chance or whether they indicate that samples are derived from different populations. The method by which these probabilities are calculated are as follows. If a sample statistic, such as the mean, of a large number of samples taken from a single population is plotted, the frequency distribution produced is known as a sampling distribution. Sampling distributions can be, and have been, produced for most statistics calculated from a sample. The production of sampling distributions is not an empirical exercise as they are derived theoretically and hence can be tabulated with precision; such tables are available for most sample statistics.

In order to use inferential statistics the researcher has to think in terms of frequency distributions and their summary statistics, as these form the basis of the sampling distributions by which results can be compared and judged. This is especially so when a decision has to be made as to whether a result is genuinely different from that expected under a given hypothesis, or whether it has occurred by chance. (Note: all sampling distributions are probability distributions as the area under any sampling distribution curve can be expressed as unity and the proportion beneath any part of the curve can then be converted into a percentage of unity and reported as a probability value.)

Null hypothesis

Research is undertaken in response to questions and the researcher has to provide possible answers. These are in the form of hypotheses, which are suggested explanations that can be tested by surveys or experiments (Chapters 12 and 13). The hypothesis under test is usually known as the null hypothesis because it is usually formulated to test that no real difference is tenable. If as a result of the tests undertaken, the null hypothesis is accepted, this means that one accepts that the changes that have taken place in the dependent variable are consistent with the hypothesis under test. If the null hypothesis is not accepted this means that either there is insufficient evidence to accept the null hypothesis, i.e. too small a sample, or that the changes in the dependent variable are not consistent with the hypothesis under test. Hence if the null hypothesis is not accepted, either one must do further tests using larger samples, or one must do further tests using a different or alternative hypothesis. If an alternative hypothesis is chosen, then this becomes the null hypothesis for future tests and should be formulated into a 'no real difference from' for the purpose of undertaking significance testing (see Chapter 11). In some cases an experiment can be designed, whereby a null hypothesis is tested directly against an alternative hypothesis, if the null hypothesis is rejected the alternative hypothesis is accepted. For example, when testing a null hypothesis that a drug produces no effect, against an alternative hypothesis that it does produce some effect.

The criteria used to accept or not accept the null hypothesis depends on the relative importance placed by the researcher on accepting or not accepting a given result as 'true'. This matter is dealt with more fully on p. 104 where Type I and Type II errors are discussed in detail. (Note: hypothesis testing is used when one wishes to test certain theories: it must not be confused with investigations designed for estimation of the size of an effect. In the latter, confidence limits (p. 87) are used, rather than significance testing.) The magnitude of the evidence may be overwhelming, but one must be sure that the results are applicable to the population from which the sample or samples are drawn. The following paragraphs on probability and confidence intervals consider two ways in which the results can be reported. The former indicates the likelihood of a result occurring by chance and the latter, the range within which the population value would lie for any chosen degree of certainty. The subject of hypothesis testing is dealt with more fully in the next chapter, where other types of error are also discussed.

Significance and probability

The decision as to whether an improbable result has occurred or whether a real difference exists, is not a simple one and depends on many factors. Inferential statistics help in being able to assign a probability to the occurrence of a result under any given hypothesis, but the researcher still has to decide whether or not to accept or reject the result as being real. If the researcher is too enthusiastic and accepts minor variations as important, this may give rise to a good deal of unproductive exploration, on the other hand if the researcher is too conservative or sceptical, this may stifle research. It is for this reason that general guidelines have come into use to help researchers, and it has become a convention that a result is accepted as statistically significant (i.e. real) if the probability of its being due to chance (if the hypothesis being tested is true) is less than 5 per cent (one in 20); highly significant if less than 1 per cent (one in a 100), and very highly significant if less than 0.1 per cent (one in a 1000). Though it must be borne in mind that when one uses these guidelines with a large number of samples (i.e. when a large number of tests are being carried out) it is to be expected that one result in 20 will be 'significant', one result in a 100 will be 'highly significant', and one result in a 1000 will be 'very highly significant' even when no such difference exists. So that when carrying out 20 or more tests, care must be taken to allow for these chance occurrences. It must also be noted that the levels of significance refer only to statistical significance and not necessarily to practical significance. Thus a result may be statistically 'highly significant' but have no practical value, because the differences noted are too small to be of any practical use. However, if the result is not statistically significant, no matter how large or important the result may seem practically, one cannot take it as being 'real' without further tests. Another important factor is to be kept in mind when using significance testing, is that the accepted levels of significance must be set before testing begins otherwise the researcher could bias his or her judgement, and possibly draw false conclusions.

As noted above, general guidelines have been laid down for application in most cases. However, the researcher has to make up his or her own mind as to what level of significance is acceptable. For example if research is being carried out on the effect of certain treatments and the treatment under test could be potentially harmful, more stringent limits will be needed than if the treatment is not potentially harmful. This is because acceptance of a potentially dangerous treatment as being effective when it is not, is likely to be more damaging than the rejection of such a treatment when it is actually beneficial. A significant find implies that it cannot reasonably be attributed to chance and thus that it deserves more attention. Note that as the required level of certainty increases, so the percentage level of significance decreases, i.e. the probability of its occurring by chance is less (probability and chance are further considered in Chapter 11).

Standard error and confidence intervals

Sampling distributions have their own mean and standard deviation but whereas the best estimate of the mean of a sampling distribution is the mean of any individual sample, the best estimate of the standard deviation of a sampling distribution is not the standard deviation of an individual sample (though it can be derived from it). In general the standard deviation of a sampling distribution is less than the standard deviation of any one individual sample. This standard deviation of the sampling distribution is known as the standard error. In particular the standard error of the sampling distribution of the mean is related to the standard deviation of the samples by the formula:

$$\text{se}\,(\bar{x}) = \frac{s}{n^{\frac{1}{2}}}$$

where s = standard deviation of the sample.

se $(\bar{x})$ = standard error of the mean.

n = number of individuals in the sample.

The fact that the sampling error of the mean is smaller than the standard deviation of an individual item, means that significance testing of the mean is far more effective than the significance testing of individual items, and that the *confidence limits* around the mean are far tighter than around any individual item. (Note: confidence limits are the limits within which a given statistic or value will lie with any given probability. So that the confidence limits of x are $x \pm t(\text{SD})$. Where x is the given statistic, SD is the standard deviation of the statistic, and t is the interval of the sampling distribution that gives rise to the chosen probability: for example for any normally distributed statistic the 95 per cent confidence limits in a large sample are $x \pm 1.96$ SD and the 99.9 per cent limits are $x \pm 3.075$ SD. The area between the two confidence limits is known as the confidence interval. It should be noted that some statisticians only refer to confidence limits or confidence intervals as the limits of the interval within which the population parameter is assumed to lie with any given degree of certainty, but for practical purposed the above definition will suffice.) The ability to make probability statements depends on the fact that in most sampling distributions, and especially the normal distribution, probabilities are fixed solely by the distance from the mean of the distribution, as measured in standard deviations. Thus, for any given probability, the smaller the standard deviation (i.e. the standard error) the smaller the distance from the mean in terms of the actual variate.

Two important statistical concepts have been used in the above line of reasoning. The first is that statistics derived from a number of samples have a given distribution, even though the measurements from which they are derived do not themselves come from that shaped distribution. This is especially so in the case of the normal distribution, because for large samples, i.e. more than 50, the sampling distribution of most statistics is virtually normal. The second concept is that standard errors can be calculated from a single sample rather than from the mean of multiple samples as described above. This is because all samples chosen at random from a given parent population have the same standard deviation, in fact all tests involving more than one sample must first establish that this is true before proceeding to significance testing. Thus the standard error or the mean of a sample is calculated from the standard deviation of that sample by dividing by the square root of the number of observations in the sample. Note, however, that the standard error of the mean applies only to the mean of the sample and not to its individual members.

Main types of sampling distribution

Statistical inference is possible because of the possibility of deriving, calculating, and tabulating sampling distributions. For most statistics derived from samples of 50 or more, the use of the normal distribution is appropriate, however, for small samples, i.e. those less than 50, this is not the case and other distribution have been derived which must be used.

In general there are six main sampling distributions used in research. These are the normal, t, F, chi-squared, binomial, and Poisson distributions. The first four distributions are all continuous distributions, i.e. there are no set intervals to the variate. The last two are discrete distributions, i.e. they deal with variates which are noncontinuous and take only particular values. Although the derivation of these distributions is beyond the scope of this book, because of their importance in medical research, brief descriptions of their main characteristics are given below:

(1) The normal distribution

The normal distribution is used to test individual values coming from a normal distribution and values of other statistics from large samples. This is especially important in the case of the mean. The normal distribution is a symmetrical bell-shaped curve and approximates to many of the distributions found in the natural world and biology. It can be regarded as the limiting form of the binomial distribution where the number of observations is infinite providing the probability of an event occurring does not become very small. Its use in statistical theory is important for the following main reasons:

(a) its properties are easy to handle mathematically;

(b) it approximates to many distributions found in nature and also to many sampling distributions;

(c) non-normal highly complicated curves can often be transformed to normal form.

Tables of the normal distribution have been extensively tabulated and published.

(2) The *t* distribution

The *t* distribution is used to test differences between means of different samples where sample size is less than 50. The chief use of the *t* distribution is in testing for differences of means in small samples from a normal population. It is a non-normal distribution defined as the distribution of the sample statistic

$$t = \frac{(\bar{x} - m) \cdot n^{\frac{1}{2}}}{s}$$

where $\bar{x}$ is the sample mean
  m is the population mean
  s is the SD of the sample
  n is the number in the sample

Note that when the observations follow a normal distribution, as n increases the *t* distribution tends to a normal distribution. Hence in large samples, testing for means can be done by using the normal distribution.

(3) The *F* distribution

The *F* distribution is used to test differences between variances of different samples. It is mainly used to test whether two sample variances come from the same population.

It is the distribution of the sample statistic:

$$F = \frac{s_1^2}{s_2^2}$$

where : $s_1^2 = S_1^2/(n_1 - 1)$
$s_2^2 = S_2^2/(n_2 - 1)$

S = sum of squares and s_1 is always greater than s_2
n_1 = number of observations in sample 1
n_2 = number of observations in sample 2.

Tables of both *t* and *F* have been extensively published for a wide number of degrees of freedom (see p. 92).

(4) The chi-squared distribution

The chi-squared distribution is used mainly to test differences between observed frequencies and their expected values. The distribution is mainly used as a test of goodness of fit or for testing independence in contingency tables. It is based on the distribution of the following sample statistic:

$$\text{Chi squared} = \sum_i \left[\frac{(A_i - E_i)^2}{E_i} \right]$$

Where A_i is the actual frequency occurring in the ith cell, E_i is the expected frequency of the ith cell, and the summation takes place over all cells. (Note: when using the chi-squared test for goodness of fit care must be taken to calculate the correct number of degrees of freedom. Whereas in the t, and F tests the only constraint is usually the grand total, in the chi-squared test the number of constraints increases by the number of statistics estimated from the sample in order to calculate the expected values: for example in calculating expected values of a normal distribution both the mean and standard deviation need to be estimated from the sample, hence the number of constrains is three, i.e. the grand total, the mean, and the standard deviation.)

When calculating chi-squared from a contingency table the number of constraints is determined by the number of columns and rows and the degrees of freedom are obtained by multiplying the number of rows minus one by the number of columns minus one, i.e. if the number of rows is r and the number of columns is c the number of degrees of freedom is $(r - 1) \cdot (c - 1)$.

The values of chi-squared have been extensively tabulated and published for a large number of probability levels and degrees of freedom.

(5) The binomial distribution

The binomial distribution is used where each event has the same probability of occurrence, and is akin to the normal distribution in the continuous case. It is a discrete distribution which enables one to calculate the chance of a given number of successes occurring in a number of trials (samples) when the probability of success at each trial is known and is constant over all trials, i.e. if the chance of success is known and constant then the binomial distribution can be used to calculate the chance of obtaining 1,2,3,4,5 . . . n successes in a sample of n.

It should be noted that the mean of a binomial distribution is np with SD $= (npq)^{1/2}$

where p = chance of success
     q = chance of failure $= (1 - p)$
     n = number in sample.

Note that as n tends to infinity the binomial distribution tends to the normal distribution. As a corollary of the above the binomial distribution allows the probability of any number of events occurring to be calculated and hence it can be used in the same way as any other probability distribution. Tables of the binomial distribution have been published but are not so widely available as the other distributions discussed.

(6) The Poisson distribution

The Poisson distribution is used where the probability of any event occurring is extremely small. It is another limiting form of the binomial distribution but in this case when the chance of success tends to zero as n tends to infinity, so that $np =$ constant. In this case the mean number of success is np with SD = $(np)^{1/2}$. Like the binomial distribution, tables of the Poisson distribution have been published and should be used whenever the chance of a success is small. Illustrations of the use of all the above distributions are given in Chapter 11.

Distributions, formulae and tables

Because distributions play a central role in statistical analysis these paragraphs bring together the various features already described concerning their use. A *distribution* is an ordered set of measurements, in which each value of the variable has a given frequency. Distributions may take many forms, but the most frequently occurring one in most branches of science is the symmetrical bell-shaped distribution known as the normal distribution.

A *population distribution* is the distribution of the measurements of all the members of a given population. However, as the whole population is not usually available for measurement, for example because the population is infinite, hypothetical, or would cost too much to measure, the population distribution is usually estimated from the *sample distribution*. This is the distribution of the measurements of the members of a sample taken from the population. A *sampling distribution*, which is not the same and must not be confused with a sample distribution, is a theoretically derived distribution of a given statistic from a given population. It can also be estimated by taking a large number of random samples from the given population. Such theoretically derived distributions have been calculated and tabulated for nearly all sample statistics.

Naturally occurring events often follow specific shaped distributions: the most common of which are the normal (for continuous variables), the binomial (for discrete variables), and the Poisson (for continuous or discrete variables where the chance of occurrence is very small). Values of sampling distributions are tabulated in terms of their probability and this allows the likelihood of obtaining any particular value of the statistic being calculated to be looked up in the appropriate statistical table.

The shape of any theoretical distribution can be described by a specific mathematical formula and statistical tests may be regarded as methods of transforming the data from one of more sets of observations into a form in which they can be compared with a known theoretical distribution or with each other. The probability of the results of those comparisons are then determined by looking up the appropriate table.

Regular use of common statistics, such as chi-squared, t, and F (see p. 88) enables the researcher to gain an impression as to whether a result is likely to be significant, even before undertaking an analysis, but references to the tables is obligatory in all circumstances. Other factors which have to be taken into account when looking up a statistical value in the table of its sampling distribution are: whether a one- or two tailed test is being used (p. 106), and the number of degrees of freedom (see below). The latter is linked with the number of measurements taken and the specific test used.

The rules pertaining to each test must be learned from textbooks or other sources, and must be adhered to all circumstances. The objectives of each test are the same: i.e. to decide whether or not a given result is consistent with the hypothesis under test. This is done by finding out from the tables of the appropriate sampling distribution the probability of its occurring by chance and then using pre-set confidence levels to decide whether or not to say such a result is a chance finding. (Note: on *degrees of freedom*. Calculations of a statistic are derived from a sample and are dependent on the number of observations in that sample. In order to avoid bias in this calculation of the statistic, the number of observations has to be reduced by one for each constraint put on the sample number, the number remaining after all the restraints have been accounted for is known as the degrees of freedom. In general most sample statistics have only one constraint (the grand total) and in these cases the number of degrees of freedom is one less than the number in the sample, i.e. $(n - 1)$. The concept of degrees of freedom is most important in small samples, i.e. those with less than 50 observations, and if not used in these circumstances can lead to serious error).

Statistical significance and practical significance

A research worker must never make decisions based purely on statistical significance. A clear distinction has to be drawn between statistical significance and practical relevance, and much outside information and knowledge has to be taken into account before the latter can be decided. This process, however, only works one way, i.e. if a result is statistically significant, it may not be of practical use. On the other hand, however large or important the result may seem, if it is not statistically significant, no conclusions can be made about its practical significance—further tests on larger samples have to be made if the researcher still believes the proposed hypothesis.

The use of significance testing is entirely dependent on the fact that the samples from which decisions are made are absolutely free from bias and have been drawn in such a way as to make them completely free from any subjective ideas of the researcher. Furthermore, the design of the experiment must be such that it is completely free from bias, and must be such that it enables the researcher to draw general conclusions.

Any restriction on the population from which samples are drawn restricts the generality of the results and it is important to recognize this fact before an experimental design is finalized. Significance testing can be a valuable tool in research but it has to be remembered that, as with most things, it can only work when it is based on sound inputs, and a well-constructed and well-executed experimental design.

The size of sample, as well as its unbiasedness, is also important, and sample sizes can sometimes be too large as well as too small. This is because if a sample size is very large, even a very small effect of no practical significance, will be statistically highly significant. For instance, an increase in survival of one day after treatment of a malignant disease may be shown to be statistically highly significant. Conversely, increased survival of 1–2 year's may not reach significance because of wide variation of sample results: i.e. genuine differences can be masked by such sample variations. Confidence intervals, which determine the limits within which the true size of the effect is likely to lie in the population, are a useful complementary tool to significance values. Thus testing for statistical significance allows the researcher to state, under the hypothesis being tested and, provided the experimental design is compatible, the probability of the observed difference occurring by chance. The researcher then has to decide the practical value of the finding.

Summary

1. Interpretation of the results of surveys and experiments involves estimating population characteristics from sample statistics.

2. Each statistic has a theoretically derived sampling distribution and the values and percentage points of each of these sampling distributions have been calculated and tabulated.

3. Changes in the dependent variable are tested using the null hypothesis.

4. The probability of a sample value derived for a statistic representing the population value, is obtained by looking up the appropriate statistical table.

5. Any result that has less than a 1 in 20 chance of arising purely by sampling variation is usually accepted as being 'significant' but this varies according to circumstances and has to be determined by the researcher *before* research commences.

6. The variation of a sample statistic can be used to determine confidence intervals between which the population parameter is assumed to lie with any given degree of certainty.

7. There are six main types of sampling distribution used in statistical testing of research. These are, the normal distribution, the *t* distribution (averages), the *F*

distribution (variances), the chi-squared distribution (expectations), the binomial distribution (fixed probability), and the Poisson distribution (extremely small probabilities).

8. Clinical and other decisions must not be made on the basis of statistical significance alone. Other sources and kinds of information must be taken into account in order to make sensible as well as ethical decisions.

9. If a statistical test proves nonsignificant, no decision as to practical significance can be taken without further tests. Whereas, if a statistical test does prove to be significant, it is up to the researcher to establish practical significance.

11. Statistical testing

Overview

This chapter considers how research questions or hypotheses can be tested. These tests are undertaken on samples and are used to assess the reliability with which sample results can be applied to the population about which the questions were posed. A student often finds it possible to follow examples in a textbook and appreciate how statistical tests match data. Yet the tests still do not seem to match the data produced in their own investigations. Two prime reasons exist for this discrepancy; firstly, as well as the requirements of core knowledge and understanding principles, time and practical experience are required to be able to group and compare data with confidence. The second reason is that statistical tests should not be produced at the end of a survey or experiment to try to match the data, rather the surveys and experiments must be designed in a specific format to ensure they comply to the requirements of a specific statistical test, this being chosen at the beginning and not the end of an investigation. The tests used depend on the type of investigation and the characteristics of the population. If the population is known or assumed to have a specific distribution, such as the normal, tests known as parametric tests should be applied (note: parametric tests are those which involve estimation of the parameters of the parent population). If this is not so, nonparametric tests, i.e. those which do not involve population parameters but other characteristics, such as the shape and density of the population distribution, are required. Other factors which have to be taken into account in statistical tests are the number of parameters which have to be estimated, and whether the results can be in either direction or limited to one end of the sampling distribution (i.e. whether a one- or two-tailed test is applied—see p. 106). Statistical tests can be categorized into tests of association, tests determining the parameters of a population from a single sample, and tests that determine whether there are any differences between two or more samples. Figures 11.1 to 11.6 provide one possible scheme for selecting the appropriate test. Tests can only provide an indication of how likely a sample result reflects what would happen in the population from which the sample is believed to be drawn. They are subject to error. The researcher has to determine what size of error is acceptable in the chosen investigation. The test and the level of significance must be chosen before starting an investigation. Significance, however, is not synonymous with practical relevance and the researcher must not be dictated to by statistical findings. Once the statistical analysis has been completed the researcher is then in a position to judge the scientific, and practical as opposed to the statistical, relevance of a finding.

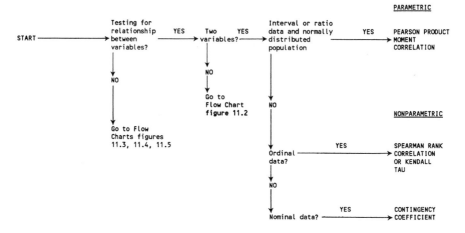

Fig. 11.1 Selecting a test for a statistical relationship between two variables.

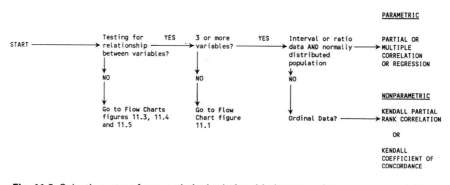

Fig. 11.2 Selecting a test for a statistical relationship between three or more variables.

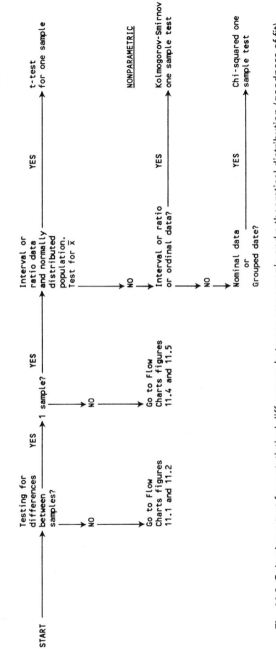

Fig. 11.3 Selecting a test for a statistical differences between one sample and a theoretical distribution (goodness of fit).

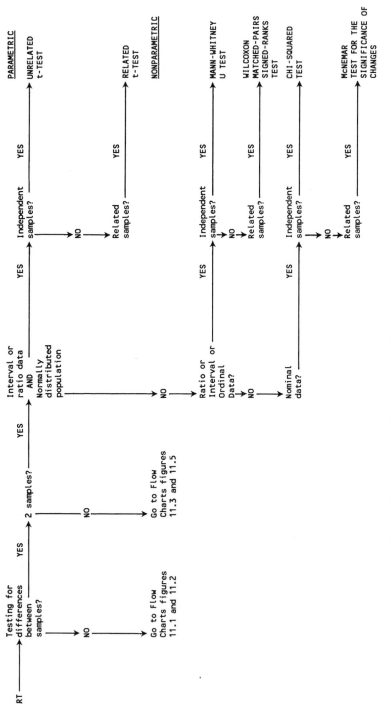

Fig. 11.4 Selecting a test for statistical differences between two samples.

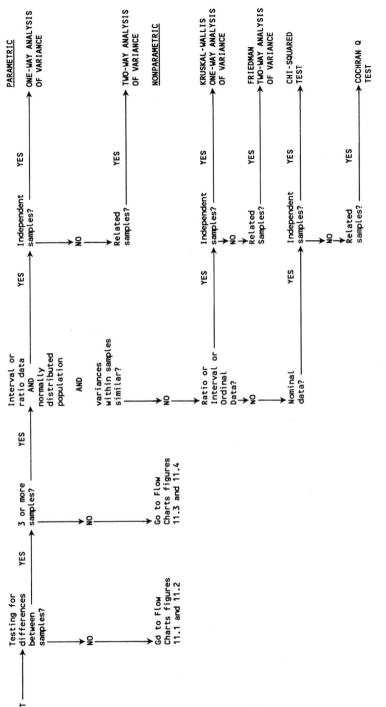

Fig. 11.5 Selecting a test for a statistical difference between three or more samples.

Fig. 11.6 OVERVIEW OF STATISTICAL TESTS

Level of Measurement	Type	One sample goodness of fit	Difference between two samples		Difference between three or more samples		Relationship between two variables
			Independent	Related	Independent	Related	
Ratio or Interval	Parametric Grouped Data	Chi squared	Unrelated t-test	Related t-test	Parametric One-way Analysis of Variance	Parametric Two-way Analysis of Variance	Pearson Product Moment Correlation
Ordinal	Non-parametric	Kolmogorov-Smirnov	Mann-Whitney U	Wilcoxon	Kruskal-Wallis one-way Analysis of Variance	Friedman Two-way Analysis of Variance	Kendall Tau or Spearman Rank Correlation
Nominal	Non-parametric	Chi-squared	Chi-squared	McNemar	Chi-squared	Cochran Q	Contingency Coefficient

Formulating hypotheses (see also Chapter 10, p. 85)

Research is undertaken in response to a question, for example what causes an event or effect; how, why, when, or where it occurs. The researcher starts off by suggesting an appropriate answer and examining how well this 'hypothesis' conforms to the observed events. In order to do this the question must first be broken down into specific measurable components, i.e. defining the factors of interest (dependent variable) and other factors (independent variables) that influence it. The problems of defining the dependent and independent variables were considered in relation to a new food product, KPH (p. 5). Similar problems are encountered in all branches of science: consider for example such extremes as identifying causative factors for earthquakes and diseases.

In any investigation the researcher is examining either the extent to which measurable changes in the dependent variable are associated with measurable changes in the independent variable(s); or the researcher is examining whether any changes take place in the dependent variable in those situations where the suggested causative factor is present or not. (Note: although the word 'causative' is used as describing the independent variable, a statistical test can only show association and is not proof of causation. In the second form of examination, the proposed answer is not always a precise measurement of the extent of a relationship but can be a qualitative answer indicating whether any changes of any sort have taken place.)

Hypothesis testing

The relationship between the chosen variables is examined either by surveying naturally occurring events or by undertaking experiments in which the researcher controls one or more of the independent variables. In any experiment the researcher can only examine part (a sample) of any population and must therefore ensure that the chosen sample is representative of the population from which it is drawn. Statistical hypotheses are statements about populations. The process of assessing the probability of any hypothesis in the light of sample evidence is called a *statistical test*. Reaching a conclusion about population characteristics on the basis of sample evidence, requires effective use of the information in the sample; different combinations of sample measurements give different kinds and amounts of information about the population. Sample measurements are used to compute a single number, called the *test statistic* which summarizes the evidence. There are essentially three quantities that enter into a statistical test:

1. the size of any real change which the test is trying to measure;

2. the size of the sample;

3. the amount of random variation in the population under investigation.

All three quantities have an influence on the design of the experiment being undertaken as the size of the sample has an effect on the sampling error, which is in turn related to the random variation in the population. The size of the sampling error affects the ability to make a decision as to the genuineness or not of the sample result, by which changes in the population are being measured. The smaller the effect being measured, the smaller needs to be the sampling error and hence the larger needs to be the size of the sample. The art of a good test design is to balance these three quantities in such a way that optimal information is obtained from a sample. This is especially important where cost considerations or restraints come into play. When testing a given hypothesis (note the hypothesis under test is generally know as the null hypothesis, as opposed to any alternative hypotheses which is under consideration), it is important to remember three things. Firstly, the greater the change shown by an experiment, the greater is the likelihood of showing a 'real effect'. The reverse is also true, viz: the smaller the change shown, the less is the likelihood of showing it to be 'real'. Secondly, the smaller the random or sampling error, the more likely it is to demonstrate a 'real effect', and the reverse—the larger the random or sampling error, the less likely it is to demonstrate a 'real' effect. Thirdly, the size of the sample determines the size of the sampling error and hence the larger the sample the more likely it is to show genuine effects and vice versa, the smaller the sample the less likely it is to show genuine or real effects.

Most statistical tests follow a similar basic reasoning whatever their design. A test value is calculated for the statistic under consideration and then by using its sampling distribution table (see p. 91), the probability of its occurrence is calculated and checked against the significance levels agreed by the researcher before commencing the experiment (see p. 86). If the probability of its occurrence is less than that set as significant, i.e. it is unlikely to have occurred by chance, the researcher concludes that the effect is 'real' and the null hypothesis, i.e. the hypothesis under test, is rejected. On the other hand if the probability of its occurrence is larger than the limits set, the researcher has no alternative but to accept the null hypothesis. One concludes that in this particular experiment there is no statistical evidence to support the hypothesis that no 'real' change has occurred that is inconsistent with the null hypothesis. The latter is true however large the change may have been. If the researcher is still convinced that a real change has occurred, the experiment must be redone using a larger sample, reducing the sampling error by which the change was judged. In all cases the researcher must remember that decisions are being made on the basis of probabilities and that there is always a chance that one might accept a 'real' effect as true, when in fact it is false, or one might reject a 'real' effect when it is 'true'. Therefore, care must be taken, when undertaking experiments, to determine whether an effect is 'real' or 'false', that one does not fall into the trap of accepting or rejecting only favourable evidence.

Every test makes certain assumptions about the populations from which the samples are drawn and the large number of available tests are a reflection of the specific requirements of various experimental designs. Figures 11.1 to 11.6 are intended as a preliminary guide to choosing a test for each experimental situation.

Statisticians differ in their choice of test and the flow charts are only one of many possible alternatives. Some of these routes are commonly used, whereas others are unusual and complex. Before commencing any research the researcher must discuss the matters with a qualified statistician. (Note; it cannot be stressed strongly enough that the need for this discussion has to be at the time of designing a study, rather than just seeking statistical help at the time of analysis.)

Statistical tests

Statistical test can be divided into tests of association, tests of goodness of fit and tests of difference.

1. Tests of association

These use correlation and/or regression techniques, for example in the KPH example one was looking for an association between KPH and energy levels, whilst in other examples one was looking for factors associated with earthquakes or disease. If the degree of correlation is found to be significant, it is suggestive that the proposed factors are the proposed causative agents, but it must again be emphasized that correlation and causation are *not* synonymous, as other unidentifiable factors could be influencing 'both events'. Emphasis has so far been given to identifying a single independent and a single dependent variable that can be measured. However, it may not be possible to separate two or more suggested independent factors or an association may be suspected between two or more independent variables and the dependent variable. Statistical tests exist for examining these multiple correlation situations, whether examining a variable in two or more samples, or the inter-relation of two or more variables within a single sample. Further tests, known as tests of regression, are used to calculate how much one value varies with another; this can be used to 'predict' one value from another.

2. Tests of goodness of fit

A single sample may be used to estimate the parameters of the population from which it is drawn. The tests may use means or proportions, they compare sample results with hypothetical or expected values. For example: the t test for small samples compares the sample mean with the expected population mean (see p. 89); the chi-squared test of goodness of fit compares the frequency of occurrence of different values of a variate against their expected values. Other tests compare the relation of various sample statistics to those expected from a normal distribution; or, when dealing with proportions, the relation to a binomial distribution. These tests are known as tests of goodness of fit, as they assess how reliably the sample result fits a hypothetical population value.

3. Statistical tests of difference

In these tests, a test statistic is used to examine the significance between the different effect of two independent variables on a dependent variable. Usually this is done by using two samples, but in a crossover design (see p. 144) both independent variables are assessed on the same sample. Further tests exist to examine the difference in effect of three or more independent variables on a dependent variable. In addition different test statistics are used for independent and related samples, i.e. whether in the experimental design members of different samples were matched or paired with each other (pp. 145–8).

Errors

In statistical testing of hypotheses there are two types of error. Type I (also known as an error of the first kind, an alpha error, or a false positive). This type of error occurs when a true hypothesis is rejected as being false. Type II (also known as an error of the second kind, a beta error, or a false negative). This type of error occurs when a false hypothesis is accepted as being true. The statistician's answer is often expressed in terms of probability (p. 86). It is up to the researcher and statistician to decide the probability level at which a hypothesis should be accepted or rejected. It must, however, be remembered that when aiming for a 95 per cent degree of certainty, a Type I error, i.e. rejecting a true hypothesis, will still occur by chance once in every 20 experiments. The researcher sets the number of acceptable errors, i.e. the probability of making a Type I error. In biomedical terms reducing Type I errors increases the specificity of a test to pick up only real effects. This argument is sound, as far as it goes. The trouble is that the researcher is not taking into account the second kind of risk, i.e. that of accepting a hypothesis when it is false (a Type II error). In biomedical terms, increasing Type II errors decreases the sensitivity of the test to pick up real effects.

Unfortunately, the chances of making Type I errors and Type II errors are inversely related (see Fig. 11.7). A balance has to be struck between these two kinds of error. The researcher has to select the level of significance appropriate for the investigation in hand. It may be important, for example not to miss any beneficial effect of a drug in a serious disease. Whereas a potentially harmful drug would have to have a very marked benefit to be used in nonserious conditions.

Increasing the specificity in picking up *only* real effects reduces the sensitivity of picking up *all* real effects: specificity is inversely related to sensitivity. Translating this into statistical terms:

Reducing the probability of Type I errors, i.e. of rejecting an hypothesis when it is true, *increases* the probability of Type II errors i.e. of accepting an hypothesis when

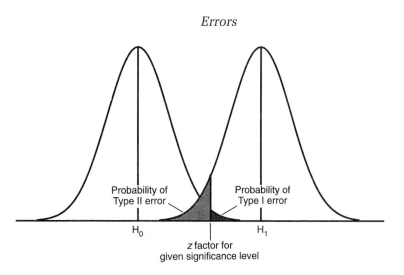

Fig. 11.7 Relationship between Type I and Type II errors. Note: (i) if the significance level is reduced, the probability of a Type I error is reduced, but the probability of a Type II error is increased. (ii) if the variance of the distributions is reduced and/or the difference between H_0 and H_1 is increased, the probability of a Type II error is reduced. (iii) H_0 is the hypothesis being tested and H_1 is an alternative hypothesis.

it is false. When calculating a statistic the researcher states the desired level of significance and, in so doing, the probability of rejecting a true hypothesis. If the researcher wants a sensitive test that will pick up more real effects, and is not too concerned about accepting 'nonreal' effects, the level of significance is reduced. Thus the probability of making a Type I error is set by the investigator and is called the level of significance. The higher the level of significance (i.e. the more extreme the finding when compared against a given hypothesis), the smaller the probability of rejecting true hypotheses, but the larger the probability of accepting false hypotheses.

For any particular test statistic, the probability of making a Type II error is a complex function of: the level of significance, whether a one- or two-tailed test is used (see below), sample size, and the actual value of the parameter of interest. In practice, it is difficult to compute Type II errors. When, therefore, the decision is taken not to reject an hypothesis, the researcher does not know the probability of being wrong: it is for this reason a nonsignificant result should be expressed as nonrejection of the hypothesis, rather than its acceptance. The *power* of a test (1-Type II error), is probability of rejecting an hypothesis when it is false, that is, the test's sensitivity to picking up genuine effects. Power is related to the size of the true effect, the particular statistical test used and also the direction of an alternative hypothesis; for a given level of probability a one-tailed test is more powerful than a two-tailed test (see below). The power of a statistical test also increases with sample size. In many practical problems, the 5 per cent or 1 per cent levels of significance strike the right balance and are usually refereed to as 'significant' and 'highly significant' respectively (p. 86). The researcher must not, however, be dictated to by convention and the significance level should be chosen according to circumstances and after discussion with the statistician.

One- and two-tailed regions of rejection

As referred to in the previous section, the points on the sampling distribution at which the researcher concludes that a result could not be caused by sampling variation alone, are usually taken as the extreme 5 per cent or 1 per cent of measurements. Thus if a result lies on or outside these points it is said to be statistically significant. In the case of a one-sided test this is illustrated in Fig. 11.8 where a cut-off point has been drawn whereby all values of the statistic lying outside this limit only account for 5 per cent of the population. For a two-sided test the extreme 5 per cent of the population is usually divided equally between the two ends of the distribution, i.e. 2.5 per cent at each tail, this is illustrated in Fig. 11.9. In this case the null hypothesis is stated without direction, for instance: 'changes in level of intake of KPH are associated with changes in a puppy's energy level', whether this energy level be greater of less than before the intake of KPH.

If the hypothesis had been stated with a direction, for instance, puppies' energy level is improved with the intake of KPH, the region of rejection would have been in just one tail of the sampling distribution as shown in Fig. 11.8. Thus the location, but not the size, of the rejection region has changed. Hence, where a difference from an hypothesis in one direction may have real consequences for practical action, but a difference in the other direction does not, a one-tailed test should be

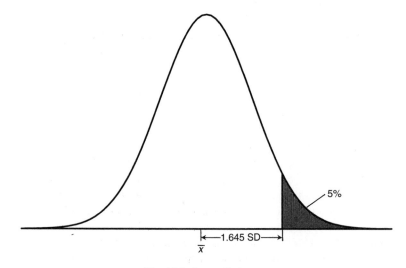

$\overline{x}$ |←—1.645 SD—→| 5%

Fig. 11.8 One-tailed test.

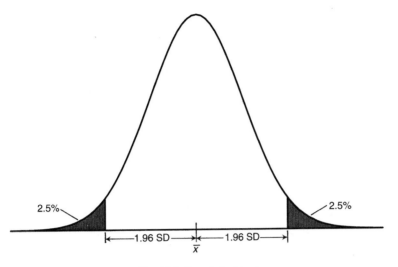

Fig. 11.9 Two-tailed test.

used. In situations where the researcher is asking 'If I do this, does it have *any* effect', a two-tailed test should be used.

Care must be taken when using statistical tables as these can be given for a one-tailed test or a two-tailed test, or both. Where a one-tailed table is given and a two-tailed test is required, one looks up *half* the required probability. If a two-tailed test is given and a one-tailed test is required, one looks up *twice* the required probability. The golden rule is always check and make sure how a table is compiled before using.

It is possible to have different levels of significance for the upper and lower tails of a distribution if it is considered important to accept or reject association at different levels of effect, for example, one may wish to be fairly certain of accepting a change if its effect reaches level (a) but have less qualms about rejecting it if its effect is less than level (b).

The number of subjects required in surveys and experiments

Research projects rarely have unlimited time, money, and resources and in planning a programme it is important to have some idea of the numbers required to demonstrate true changes between samples or between a sample and some known standard. This also has ethical considerations, not only in the appropriate use of funding, but also in the avoidance of prolonged ineffective treatment or delaying effective forms of treatment. When designing a project some knowledge of the likely number of subjects allows decisions to be made on the logistics, feasibility, practicality, and costing, and for these factors to be balanced with the desirability and the potential benefits of the research. One can not calculate the precise numbers required, this needs the results of the investigation about to be undertaken. However, a useful approximation can be obtained taking into account the various factors controlled by the investigator. Sample sizes are calculated for different magnitudes of change taking into account the inherent variation of the populations being studied.

Factors controlled by the investigator

1. The number and size of the samples.
2. If two or more samples are used, whether to use paired samples or, if independent, whether equivalent numbers should be present in each sample.
3. The statistic to be compared. This often falls into the category of a mean or a proportion.
4. Whether to use a one- or two-tailed test (see p. 106).
5. The level of probability required for detecting a difference at any given significance level, i.e. the power (1-beta) of the study and how low the chance of accepting a false hypothesis is to be.
6. The desired level of significance, i.e. the probability of rejecting a true hypothesis.

Factors depending on the true characteristics of the population(s) under study

1. The amount of inherent variation present in the parent population(s). This information may be available from previous data, or a pilot study may be required to obtain an estimate for the figure.
2. The size and/or range of possible changes. The researcher then has to decide what size of statistically significant change is to be regarded as both meaningful and important.

Numbers in a sample

The size of a sample, i.e. the number of subjects to be tested depends on two main criteria:

1. The variance of the population being sampled.
2. The size of the effect which needs to be ascertained at any given confidence level.

If the variance of the population is nil, i.e. all subjects are exactly the same, only a sample of one would be needed, as any reaction from this one subject would by definition of zero population variance apply to all the other members of the population. On the other hand if the population variance is very large in comparison to the size of effect needed to be shown a very large sample would be needed in order to achieve a reasonable degree of confidence.

As an illustration, if the mean of a sample is tested for a given size of effect at the 5 per cent level of confidence, and if the size of effect to be tested is y, it is known that (a) the standard error of the mean is SD $(pop)/n^{1/2}$ and (b) that the 5 per cent confidence level is 1.96 SD from the mean. Thus:

$$y = 1.96 \; \text{SD}(\bar{x})$$

$$y = 1.96 \frac{\text{SD} \; (pop)}{n^{\frac{1}{2}}}$$

$$y^2 = 3.8416 \frac{\text{var} \; (pop)}{n}$$

$$n = \frac{3.8416 \; \text{var} \; (pop)}{y^2}.$$

Similar formulae can be derived for any shift in the statistic being tested. However, the formula for the standard error of any statistic can sometimes be quite complicated. When in doubt, it is always better to consult a qualified statistician. Figure 11.10 gives these for a percentage at different percentage levels and for different size of samples. Thus, if the change of success was 25 per cent, and a sample of 1000 was taken, the average shift in the percentage to be significant at the 5 per cent level would need to be at least (1.96) (1.37) = 2.68. The chance of success in the sample would need to be outside 25 ± 2.68, i.e. 27.68 – 22.32 to regarded as significantly different from 25 per cent.

The chart in Fig. 11.10 has been extracted from a full set of tables prepared by Stuart.[1] To avoid using tables a nomogram has been prepared by Rosenbaum[2] and is reproduced in Fig. 11.11. Note it is often possible, by making the necessary assumptions, to adapt sample sizes for percentages to continuous variables.

Fig. 11.10 se of a chosen percentage for different sample sizes

n	p = 50%	25%	1%
25	10.00	8.66	1.99
100	5.00	4.33	0.99
500	2.24	1.94	0.44
1000	1.58	1.37	0.31
5000	0.71	0.61	0.14

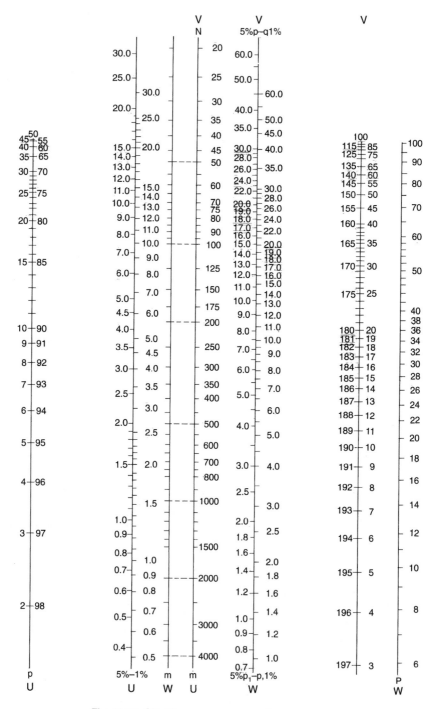

Fig. 11.11 Significance nomogram for percentages.

A significance chart for percentages

The nomogram in Fig. 11.11 is used for the solution of three distinct problems, referred to as U, V and W. Three parallel scales in the diagram are labelled with the corresponding appropriate letter, the two outer scales measuring the independent variables of percentage (p or P) and size of sample (m or N). In any problem, the straight line joining a pair of given values of these variable will cut the central scale in the required solution.

U. The scale m shows the size of the sample; the scale p shows the percentage having a specific attribute. The central scale then gives 95 per cent and 99 per cent confidence limits to p.

Example (1)

Sample size 400, of whom 30 per cent (or 70 per cent have a specific attribute: the 95 per cent confidence interval is $30 + 4.5$ per cent (or $70 + 4.5$ per cent), and the 99 per cent confidence interval is $30 + 6$ per cent (or $70 + 6$ per cent).

V. This refers to samples m and n of two populations ($N = m + n$ shown on left-hand scale), with percentage p and q of the separate samples having the same attribute ($P = p + q$ shown on the right-hand scale). The central scale gives 5 per cent and 1 per cent significance levels for the difference $p - q$.

Example (2)

For a pair of samples $N = m + n = 500$:
   (i) with $p = 16$ per cent of m, $q = 9$ per cent of n (i.e. $P = p + q$ 25);
       $p - q = 7$ which is > 5 per cent sig. and < 1 per cent sig.
  (ii) if $p = 15$ per cent, $q = 10$ per cent ($P = 25$);
       $p - q + 5$ which is < 5 per cent sig.
 (iii) if $p = 17$ per cent, $q = 8$ per cent ($P = 25$);
       $p - q = 9$ which is > 1 per cent sig.

W. The scale m shows size of sample. If $p1$ and $p2$ ($P = p1 + p2$ shown on right scale) are percentages of m, having different (mutualy exclusive) attributes, the central scale gives 5 per cent and 1 per cent significance levels for the difference $p1 - p2$.

The method used in similar to the example for V, reading m for N and $p1 - p2$ for $p - q$.

Note

1. For intermediate values not marked on the scales, it is sufficiently accurate to interpolate linearly.

2. Random sampling is assumed throughout.

3. The nomogram should not be used for small numbers, since the approximations are inaccurate.

4. In comparing two groups, fairly equal numbers should be used, this again because of the approximations used in drawing the nomograms.

5. The V and W scales tell only one side of the story. Assuming that there is no difference between groups, the chart safeguards against saying there is. But there is still a risk that a difference truly exists which is discounted. If it is important to trace such a difference, a larger sample must be taken. (It is almost axiomatic in statistics that samples need to be much larger than you think.) The emphasis in the charts is decidedly against admitting false claims.

6. Approximations used for the U scales include the asymptotic normal form for the binomial distribution, the population variance taken as the sample value and equal confidence limits. The latter is particularly inaccurate for small or large percentages.

7. Additional approximations for the V scales include the assumption of equal sample sizes, and a pooled estimate of variance.

8. The W scales also use the mean of the groups to estimate the variance, while taking account of a convariance term.

Formulate the research hypothesis

↓

Do some preliminary tests

↓

State the hypothesis to be tested

↓

Design the investigation

↓

Choose the statistical test to match the design

↓

Set the significance level

↓

Decide whether to use a one or two-tailed test

↓

Calculate the test statistic

↓

Find the critical value of the test statistic
from the relevant statistical table

↓

Compare the value of the test statistic
obtained against the critical value

↓

Decide whether to accept or reject the hypothesis being tested

Fig. 11.12 Flow chart of the stages in statistical testing.

Examples of use of statistical tests

The stages in statistical testing, incorporating the various factors considered are summarized in Fig. 11.12; also review the flow charts on the choice of statistical test (Figs. 11.1 to 11.6).

1. Tests of goodness of fit—chi-squared

In the example of a sample of blood pressure in 60 hypertensive patients (see p. 00), it is required to find out whether the sample conforms to a normal distribution. For this test use is made of the chi-squared test for goodness of fit. The mean and standard deviation have already been calculated.

$\bar{x} = 130.75$ mm/Hg

$SD = 12.58$ mm/Hg.

The expected frequencies of a normal distribution with the above mean and standard deviation is as follows:

	x	$(x - \bar{x})/SD$	Σp	P	Expected
Up to	117.5	−1.053	0.1463	0.1463	8.778
	122.5	−0.655	0.2562	0.1099	6.594
	127.5	−0.258	0.3982	0.1420	8.520
	132.5	0.139	0.5553	0.1571	9.426
	137.5	0.536	0.7040	0.1487	8.922
	142.5	0.934	0.8248	0.1208	7.248
Over	142.5	—	1.0000	0.1752	10.512
Total				1.0000	60

Σp is derived from a table of the normal probability distribution.
Note that because the chi-squared test requires a minimum expected frequency of five in each category, the end categories of the distribution on p. 70 have been combined. Also note that category limits have to take into account accuracy of measurement in this case to the nearest 5 mm/Hg. Chi-squared $= \Sigma[(A - E)^2/E]$ can now be calculated:

		Actual (A)	Expected (E)	$(A - E)^2/E$
Up to	117.5	8	8.778	0.069
	122.5	6	6.594	0.054
	127.5	8	8.520	0.032
	132.5	15	9.426	3.296
	137.5	7	8.922	0.414
	142.5	6	7.248	0.215
Over	142.5	10	10.512	0.025
Total			10.000	4.105

Chi-squared = 4.105; df = 4. (Note: there are seven cells (categories) and three constraints, i.e. the grand total, the mean and the SD of the distribution being tested, hence df = (7 − 3) = 4.) From the tables of chi-squared:

$$P\ 0.5 = 3.36;\ P\ (0.3) = 4.88;\ P\ (0.05) = 9.49$$

i.e. if the population from which these observations were taken was normal, the chance of getting a value of chi squared of 4.105 with four degrees of freedom lies between 1/3 and 1/2.

So there is no evidence to suggest that the distribution of blood pressure is other than normal. However, the relatively large difference between the actual and expected for the 130 mm/Hg category would be an indication of recording error, i.e. that recorders are rounding more than expected to 130 mm/Hg. Note in order to consider rejecting the hypothesis that the observations came from a normal distribution, chi-squared with 4df would have had to be greater than 9.49.

2. Example of use of *t* test

In the sample of 60 hypertension patients the mean of the sample was 130.75 mm/Hg with an SD of 12.58 mm/Hg. Suppose an hypothesis had been put forward that the average blood pressure level is 135 mm/Hg. Could the sample of 60 patients have come from a population with mean 135 mm/Hg. To test this hypothesis the *t* test is used:

$$t = \frac{|\bar{x}_s - u|}{SD/n^{\frac{1}{2}}}$$

where $\bar{x}_s$ is the mean of the sample
$u =$ is the mean of the population under test
SD is the sample standard deviation
n is the number of observations in the sample
degrees of freedom = $(n − 1)$

note $SD_{\bar{x}} = SD/n^{\frac{1}{2}}$.

Before carrying out the test it needs to be agreed at which level of significance the hypothesis will be accepted. For illustrative purposes the 5 per cent level will be taken. The *t* test for the sample of hypertensive patients is as follows:

$$t = \frac{|130.75 - 135|}{12.50/(60)} = \frac{4.25}{1.625} = 2.615$$

df = 60 − 1 = 59
from the *t* table $P(t)$ 5 per cent = 2.0
$P(t)$ 1 per cent = 2.66.

So that the probability of getting a value of t of 2.615 with 59 df, is just over 0.01: i.e. the probability that the sample comes from a population with mean of 135 mm/Hg is just over one in a hundred; as the 5 per cent significance level was agreed before the test, it would be concluded that the sample does not come from a population with average blood pressure of 135 mm/Hg.

3. Example of use of *F* test

Suppose a further sample of 30 hypertensive patients was taken which had a mean of 129.2 mm/Hg and a SD of 11.5 mm/Hg. Before combining the two samples it is necessary to show that they both could have come from the same parent population. To do this it is necessary to show that they both have (a) the same SD, and (b) the same mean.

To test for SD's the F test is used

$$\text{where } F = \frac{s_1^2}{s_2^2} \text{ when } s_1 > s_2.$$

In the two samples of hypertensive patients

$s_1 = 12.58$
$s_2 = 11.50$

Hence

$$F = \frac{(12.58)^2}{(11.5)^2} = 1.196$$

$df_1 = 59; df_2 = 29.$

The 5 per cent level of F for the above df is 1.39. Therefore there is no evidence to suggest that the two samples have different SD's.

The best estimate of the population SD is now therefore,

$$SD = \left[\frac{59(12.58)^2 + 29(11.5)^2}{89} \right]^{\frac{1}{2}} = 12.17 \text{ mm/H}$$

As for a comparison of the mean, the appropriate t test is:

$$t = \frac{|\bar{x}_1 - \bar{x}_2|}{s[1/n_1 + 1/n_2]^{\frac{1}{2}}}$$

$$df = (n_1 + n_2) - 2$$

i.e. for the two samples quoted above:

$$t = \frac{(130.75 - 129.2)}{12.17(1/60 + 1/30)^{\frac{1}{2}}} = \frac{1.55}{(12.17)(0.224)} = 0.57$$

$df = (60 + 30) - 2 = 88 \;\; P > 0.5$.

Thus all the evidence is consistent with the hypothesis that the two samples come from the same population with

$$\bar{x} = \frac{(130.75)60 + (129.2)30}{90} = 130.23 \text{ mm/Hg}$$

$SD = 12.17$ mm/Hg.

4. Use of the binomial and Poisson distributions

(a) The binomial distribution

If the chance of a given event occurring is p and the chance of its not occurring is $q = (1 - p)$, the expected probability of specific events occurring can be obtained form the expansion of the binomial distribution as follows:

$$(p + q)^n = p^n + np^{n-1}q + \frac{n(n-1)}{2}p^{n-2}q^2 + \binom{n}{r}p^{n-r}q^r$$

This distribution has $\bar{x}. = n \cdot p$

$$SD = (npq)^{\frac{1}{2}}.$$

Thus if the chance of an event occurring is 1/3, the average number of times it will be expected to occur in a sample of 60, is $1.3 \times 60 = 20$, with an SD of (60, 1/3. 2/3)$^{1/2} = 3.651$. Thus in a sample of 60 at the 5 per cent probability level the event could occur:

$20 \pm (1.96^*)(3.651) = 20 \pm 7.2$, i.e. between 13 and 27 without raising doubts of any bias in the sampling or on the probability of the occurrence (p), i.e. 1/3.

If proportions instead of frequencies are used:

$$\bar{x} = p$$

$$SD = \left(\frac{pq}{n}\right)^{\frac{1}{2}}.$$

*Same probability limits as $N(0.1)$ distribution.

Thus using the previous sample of 60, the expected proportion of the event occurring is 1/3, with an SD of $[(1/3)(2/3)/60]^{1/2} = 0.06085$.

For example, $0.333 \pm 1.96 \times 0.06085$
$$= 0.333 \pm 0.1193$$
$$= 0.214 + 0.453.$$

Note that when multiplying by 60, these limits are exactly the same as those given previously for frequencies.

(b) The Poisson distribution

The Poisson distribution is a limiting form of the binomial distribution when p is small and n large with $np = m$, when m is a constant. In this case the chance of r successes is $m^r e^{-m} / r!$

where e is the mathematical constant ($e \sim 2.718$). The distribution has $\bar{x} = m = np$ and $SD = m^{1/2} = (np)^{1/2}$.

An example of the use of the Poisson curve is as follows. Supposing it is known that in a town of 1 million population, on average one death per day is expected, then the probability of the number of deaths per day, based on the Poisson

Table 11.1 Probability of deaths occurring per day in a town with a population of 1 million

Number of deaths	P (Probability of occurence)	1/P (Expected number of days within which the number of deaths in Column 1 will occur)	p × 365 Expected number of days per year in which the number of deaths in Column 1 will occur)
0	0.367879	2.72	134.3
1	0.367879	2.72	134.3
2	0.183940	5.44	67.1
3	0.061313	16.31	22.4
4	0.015328	65.24	5.6
5	0.003066	326.16	1.1
6	0.000511	1957	0.2
7	0.000073	13 699	
8	0.000009	111 111	
9	0.000001	1 000 000	
10 or more	0.000001	1 000 000	
Total	1.000000		365

distribution, can be calculated or obtained from tables of the Poisson distribution. From these probabilities can be calculated the expected number of days within which a given number of deaths per day will occur once, or the expected number of days in a year in which a given number of deaths will occur (see Table 11.1).

Thus 0 or 1 deaths a day are to be expected every 2–3 days; two deaths a day every 5–6 days; three deaths a day should occur once in every 16 to 17 days; four deaths a day should occur once in every 65 days; and five deaths a day every 326 days, i.e. approximately once a year. However, six deaths will only occur once in every 1957 days, i.e. once in every 5 years. These expected frequencies can then be compared with the actual frequency of occurrence by using the chi-squared test, or warning limits can be set which if crossed, would be an indication that the average of one death per day has changed.

Summary

1. At the start of any research the researcher formulates the hypothesis to be tested. This is called the null hypothesis. After the experiments have been completed, statistical tests are carried out and the researcher either accepts or rejects the hypothesis being tested. If the hypothesis is not accepted another hypothesis has to be formulated or further tests has to be carried out, using large samples.

2. To test an hypothesis, the researcher compares the sample statistic obtained against its sampling distribution. By so doing, it is possible to state the likelihood of the value occurring if the hypothesis is true. If the likelihood is less than a given level, set by the researcher before the commencement of the test, the hypothesis is not accepted. Probability levels for determining the likelihood of an effect are usually set at 5 per cent, 1 per cent or 0.1 per cent where the smaller the probability value used the greater the degree of statistical significance that can be given to the finding.

3. Three quantities go into a statistical test (a) the size of the effect, (b) the number of measurements, i.e. the size of the sample and (c) the amount of inherent variation in the population under investigation.

4. Increasing the degree of significance (i.e. reducing the probability value) (a) increases the chance of rejecting an hypothesis when it is true. This type of error is known as Type I error, an error of the first kind, an alpha error, or a false positive, (b) reduces the chance of accepting a false hypothesis. This type of error is know as a Type II error, an error of the second kind, a beta error, or a false negative.

5. The power of a test (1 - Type II error) is the probability of rejecting an hypothesis when it is false. This means the greater the power the greater the probability of picking up real effects. Power depends on the size of the true effect, the size of the sample, the test used and the level of significance chosen.

6. For a given significance level, one-tailed tests are more discerning than two-tailed tests. In a two-tailed test of significance the hypothesis merely states that some effect exists; in a one-tailed test the direction of the effect is also predicted.

7. The numbers of subjects required in an experiment is related to the experimental design, the method of comparison, the desired level of significance, the variation of the parent population, and the size of the statistical significant change needed to be regarded as meaningful and important. Some indication of the last two factors can be obtained from a pilot study.

References

1. Stuart, A. (1963). Standard errors for percentages. *Applied Statistics*, 12, 87–101.
2. Rosenbaum, S.
   No general references to statistical methods have been given as each researcher needs to chose the books best suited to his or her needs. The following references provide some useful statistical tables. Discussion with a qualified statistician will generally help in deciding what is the best text from among the reasonably large selection available.
3. Fisher, R.A. and Yates, F. (1957). *Statistical tables*. Oliver & Boyd, Edinburgh.
4. Lindley, D.V. and Miller, J.C.P. (1962). *Cambridge elementary statistical tables*. Cambridge University Press.
5. Molina, E.C. (1942). *Poisson's exponential binomial limit*. Nostrand, New York.
6. Pearson, K. (1931). *Tables for statisticians and biometricians*. Cambridge University Press.

12. Planning and carrying out an investigation

Overview

Investigations can be conveniently subdivided into surveys and experiments. In both surveys and experiments, the researcher is attempting to answer the prime questions set out in Chapter 8: what produces an effect, what is the size of the effect, and what produces the best effect? The same statistical tests can be applied in their analysis and their results reported with a given level of confidence. The various stages of investigation and subdivision of surveys and experiments are summarized in Figs. 12.1, 12.2 and 13.1.

Design and analysis of a survey (Fig. 12.2)

Surveys comprise passive observation of naturally occurring events, interfering with these as little as possible. Their disadvantages are that the researcher is not in control of the variables and precise hypotheses cannot always be tested or valid answers always obtained. They also involve dealing with a large number of observations. When gathering data from a large number of individuals, a questionnaire is commonly used and careful attention must be given to its format; sampling techniques are also critical if one is to avoid bias. When estimating population characteristics from surveys it is useful to distinguish between descriptive techniques used for examining the characteristics of the population, and analytic techniques used when looking for relationships between these characteristics. However, this distinction is sometime blurred.

A substantial component of biomedical statistical surveys is made up of the science of *epidemiology*—the study of disease in its natural environment. The advantage of this form of study is that a large number of subjects are used and hence a better overall picture is obtained as to the cause and natural history of disease, as well as the effect of preventive programmes and treatments. Surveys also provide a good perspective of the disease in the community and the related health-care needs. Epidemiology incorporates all survey techniques, as well as having its own specific terminology and methods, such as the production of *life tables*.

Documentation

Research is concerned with seeking answers to questions. To ensure consistency, a record is needed from which to ask the questions and document the answers. One

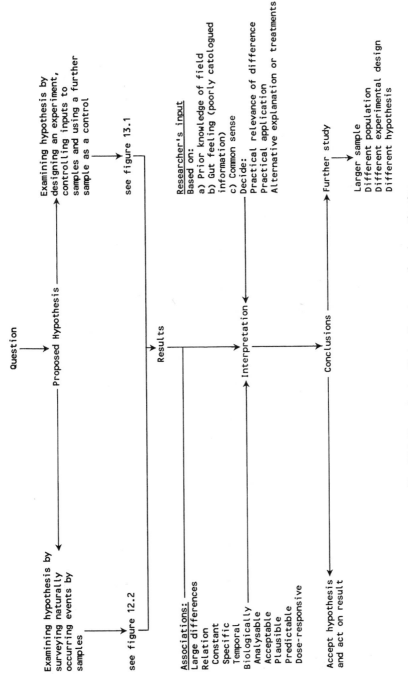

Fig. 12.1 Flow chart outlining the stages of an investigation.

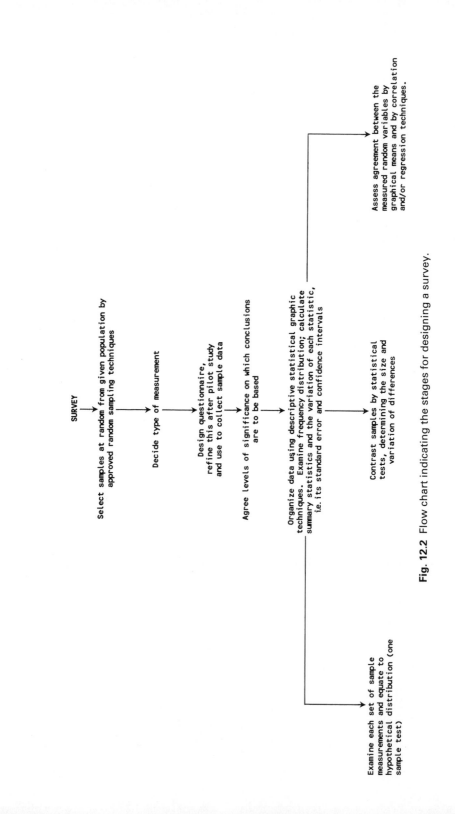

Fig. 12.2 Flow chart indicating the stages for designing a survey.

SURVEY

Select samples at random from given population by approved random sampling techniques

Decide type of measurement

Design questionnaire, refine this after pilot study and use to collect sample data

Agree levels of significance on which conclusions are to be based

Organize data using descriptive statistical graphic techniques. Examine frequency distribution; calculate summary statistics and the variation of each statistic, i.e. its standard error and confidence intervals

Contrast samples by statistical tests, determining the size and variation of differences

Assess agreement between the measured random variables by graphical means and by correlation and/or regression techniques.

Examine each set of sample measurements and equate to hypothetical distribution (one sample test)

of the first important steps, therefore, is to construct the record or questionnaire. If the questions are incomplete, ill-conceived or inadequately answered, the research will not yield reliable or valid findings. In the following paragraphs, different types of questionnaire are discussed, together with how to word them so that the answers are reliable and valid. The importance of piloting a questionnaire before use is stressed. There are numerous methods of data collection. They include the analysis of existing documents, the filling in of forms by subject or observer, and the interviewing of human subjects using a schedule or a mailed personal questionnaire. Thus the questionnaire may be completed by researcher, observers, interviewers, or by subjects themselves. The greater the number of people answering the questions, and the less their training, the greater the care that must be taken in constructing the questionnaire.

Two very widely used techniques for surveys are the *interview schedule* and the *mailed questionnaire*. In the former, although every interviewer receives the same questionnaire schedule, and although the interviewing procedure is standardized, there remain differences in the way in which questions are put to each respondent and these may have an important influence on results. The interviewer may, for instance, give an indication of opinion by the tone of voice. It is therefore important that the interviewer is trained beforehand and can be given detailed instructions to which he or she can refer. The great advantage of the interview, is that the interviewer can make sure that the respondent understands the purpose of the research and the questions being asked, thus ensuring that relevant answers are given. Above all the interviewer builds up and maintains rapport, so the respondent remains interested and responsive to the end of the interview. Interviews can be expensive in that they may include travelling, subsistence cost and payment to the interviewer, even if the interview is unsuccessful, for instance when the respondent is not available. Furthermore, interviewers have to be trained in the use of a particular questionnaire and takes time and money. The chief advantages of the mailed questionnaire are its cheapness, since it does not require field workers, and that a much larger sample can be covered for only a modest increase in cost. However, by eliminating the interviewer, the questionnaire has to be much simpler, since no additional explanations can be given. It also needs to be shorter, since without the interviewer's presence, interest is likely to wane more quickly. A mailed questionnaire cannot cover people of low intelligence or of very limited educational background. It also lacks the personal introduction of the research by the interviewer, although a good covering letter can be of great help. In general the response rate to a mailed questionnaire is much lower than that to a personal interview and this can in some cases invalidate the survey, as very low response rates are often an indication of a biased sample.

Question types

A *filter* question is used to exclude a respondent from a particular question sequence when these questions are irrelevant to that respondent. Thus, the purposes of a set of questions might be to find out about a respondent's views of KPH. The first question will be about whether the puppy has ever been fed with KPH. If the answer is negative, the respondent is instructed to miss the questions on the feeding of KPH. Broadly speaking, all questions are either *closed* or *open*. The closed question is one in which the respondent is provided with a choice of alternative replies. In open types of questions, the respondent is not given any alternatives but has to answer with a full statement. The chief advantage of open questions is the freedom it gives to the respondent, although they require more thought and are more time consuming. This type of information may also be of value to the researcher in providing the basis of new hypotheses. The difficulty with open questions is that replies have to be categorized prior to analysis, and this takes time. Often a good compromise between an open or closed question is to give a choice of alternative replies, together with a final open section, allowing respondents to add further information if they consider the choices provided are not sufficient.

Elaboration of the closed question

Ranking involves arranging the responses in order, with regard to some characteristic. The respondents, for instance, might be asked to rank a whole series of food products designed for puppies, according to the likelihood of buying each of them. Ten items are usually the most an individual can rank. Ranking provides information on the order of choice, but not on the extent of differences in preference between the ranked factors.

Ratings provide a definition of view. In the KPH example the degree of importance attached to various attributes of KPH could be found out using Table 12.1. Numerical values can be given to the judgements, for example, 'not important' being given to a value of 1, and 'very important' the value 3. The number of steps in a rating scale usually varies from 3 to 10, depending on the degree of discrimination needed. However, respondents are generally unable to make the fine discriminations asked for on a 10 point scales, except for those respondents who have extreme views and they will tend to use the extreme categories. To get around this problem,

Table 12.1 Establishing the degrees of importance puppy owners attach to various attributes of KPH

Factor	Very Important	Important	Not important
Nutritional value			
Keeps puppy very fit			
Puppy likes it			
Easy to clean utensils			
Easily obtainable			
Price			

a 10 point scale can be reduced by combining one or more categories during analysis. After deciding the number of steps in a scale, the extremes need to be defined or better still, each step defined. Most rating scales have opposites at each end, so that the middle point on the scale indicate a neutral point. For example: Puppy is very fit. Puppy is fit. Puppy is fairly fit. Puppy is a bit fit. Puppy is very unfit.

Other scales range from a neutral or zero value to an extreme value, as in the early example of a scale of importance, where the range is from not important to 'very important'. One of the difficulties with rating is the 'halo' effect; instead of giving attention to each item the respondent is influenced by an overall feeling of like or dislike. For example, if rating KPH on a series of factors, such as puppies fitness, price, and easy cleaning of utensils, the overall view about KPH will affect the ratings given for each of the different factors. Another problem is that different respondents may be making judgements against different standards: a breeder of puppies, for instance, is likely to have higher standards of fitness than many other owners.

An *index* groups together the scores attained in a series of linked questions. For instance, the answer to a series of questions about the owner's concern over their puppy's welfare could be combined into a single figure or index where a high score would indicate a great deal of concern for the puppy, whilst a low or negative score would indicate very little concern for the puppy. In general the base of an index is taken as 100 and all scores are indexed to this base so that greater than average concern would have an index above 100 whilst below average concern would have an index below 100. Note that the creation of scales and indices are not always as simple as they look and expert advice should be taken before using them in research.

Question wording

Great precision is needed in framing questions. Suppose, for example, the researcher wants to know how long a puppy has been in a household. The question 'when did you buy the puppy'? may get the response 'my Mum owns the puppy not me' whilst if the question is rephrased to 'how long have you had the puppy'? the response elicited might be 'since my last birthday''. It is important not to give the impression that the answer should be known. For instance, a question such as 'When did you first buy KPH?' assumes that the respondent knows the answer. People are often reluctant to admit that they do not know, and if they are anxious to please, may guess the answer. It is better to start with a question such as 'Can you remember when you first bought KPH?' If the answer is 'no' then they could be asked to guess whereas if the answer is 'yes' the original question on 'When did you first buy?' could be asked. It is usually better to keep questions short—preferably not more than 20 words—and to use very familiar words. Technical terms should never be used unless one is absolutely sure that they will be known to the respondents. Avoid double negatives in the sentence such as 'Would you rather not give a nonspecialized food product to your puppy?'.

Classification questions are a special type of factual question such as age, sex, marital status and income earned. They are of special significance in subdividing the sample during analysis for comparison. They should normally be at the end of a questionnaire, since they can seem very intrusive and it is better to establish a rapport first. It is important to ensure that the categories of reply do not overlap, resulting in response ambiguity. For instance, when collecting information about the age of puppies, such categories as 'under 6 months' and '6 months to under a year' should be used rather such categories as 'up to 6 months' and '6 months to a year'". An answer should be obtained for every question by including categories such as 'not known', 'no information' or 'other'. This is because no response at all is open to more than one interpretation. It could mean the respondent has missed a question, does not know, or the answer does not fit any of the categories given. The units of measurement in which a response is to be given should also be clearly given, if the reply is to be unambiguous. The method of measurement should also be given, together with the accuracy with which it should be taken.

Thought should be given as to whether an answer can be provided with sufficient accuracy for the purpose of the enquiry. Owners who buy KPH regularly will remember that they purchase it. However, those who rarely use it may not remember whether or not they have bought it within a set period. The researcher needs to weigh up the likely accuracies. Provided inaccuracies are random, their effect is unlikely to produce a trend in the data and so invalidate the results.

The researcher should also be alert to different use of categories by respondents on account of differences in opinion. This could happen when several vets are examining the same puppy and commenting on its fitness. Leading questions suggest what the answer should be. For instance, 'When did you first notice the loss of energy in your puppy?' It is also important that questions are worded neutrally and it is also important to avoid words which are emotionally 'loaded'. A different response would be obtained to the question 'Does your puppy have a good appetite?' than to the question 'Does your puppy over-eat?'.

Be aware of prestige loading in questions. If the respondent has indicated that they learned about KPH initially through a newspaper advertisement, they may be more prepared to admit to reading certain newspapers rather than others. It is also important to remember that people do not like to admit to reprehensible behaviour such as the puppy biting people. Respondents may even find some questions embarrassing, such as those asking about the sexual behaviour of the puppy. In these instances, it may be better to use a closed question where all the alternatives are set out, so that the respondent is aware that their puppy is not the only one engaging in a particular form of behaviour.

Attitude statement

An attitude is a tendency to act or react in a certain manner when confronted with certain situations. Attitudes may be reinforced by a question and often attract strong feelings that will lead to particular forms of behaviour. Attitudes may be held with greater or lesser conviction. To one person, puppies may be of passing interest, whereas to another they may be of great importance. The latter individual is more likely to agree or disagree strongly than the former to a whole series of questions dealing with the treatment of animals. Extremes of attitude (either positive or negative) are usually held with more vehemence, whereas the more neutral positions may be defended with less intensity. Some attitudes are more enduring than others. Remember that attitudes are emotional and it is important to avoid a stilted approach in writing attitude statements. The statement 'Sometimes my puppy is a nuisance' is perhaps a better statement than 'Sometimes I am too busy to pay attention to the needs of my puppy'. Since so much depends on the way the issue is put into words, a single item or a single question is often unreliable. It is better to ascertain attitude through a series of questions selected from a larger pool, based on the item's ability to differentiate during a pilot study.

The number of questions to include

It is tempting to collect as much information as possible in order to learn the maximum amount. The disadvantage of this approach is that respondents will lose interest and answer questions less accurately. Worse still, some individuals may find the length so daunting that they will decide not to take part. If a number of respondents are from a particular subgroup, for example, those not experiencing any problems or difficulties covered by the questionnaire, the results will not be representative. It is a good discipline to ask of every question; 'Is it really making a useful contribution?', 'Can I take answers from it which are sufficiently accurate for my purposes?', and 'Will I be able to analyse the results sensibly?'. One way of asking more questions, without losing interest in commitment of respondents, is to subdivide the sample into subgroups and target some of the questions on particular groups. Care must be taken, however, not to introduce bias from the choice of subgroups. A longer series of questions may be tolerated if they are closed, and on reading the question the respondent can, with minimal effort, immediately select an appropriate category.

Piloting questions

The earlier stages of pilot work are likely to be exploratory, involving lengthy unstructured interviews. From this in-depth discussion appropriate questions evolve. Pilot studies help devise the wording of questions. When a question is reworded after pilot work, it must be piloted again, since the rewording may have introduced new difficulties. To determine whether a question needs rewording the researcher examines the replies. If responses show misunderstanding, or are too vague or too limited, the question needs rewording. If respondents have difficulty answering the question, it may also be that they do not have the information required. An important use of pilot work is to turn open questions into closed ones by examining the answers given and categorizing them.

The questionnaire may go through many drafts and it is usually best to start off with a number of booklets of questions, each booklet containing a subset of the total number of questions. In this way the pilot work is broken into a number of smaller operations. Each subset is then tested by a pilot sample. The answers to each question are copied onto sheets of paper, one sheet per question. In this way, problems with particular questions can be identified quickly. Pilot respondents should be as similar as possible to those to be used in the main research, both in terms of age, relevant characteristic, education, and literary background. Letters of introduction should be piloted, as should various ways of reducing non-response. Thinking through to the analysis of the results is also an important aspect of piloting. For example, if an overall index of some factor is needed, a suitable rating scale must be devised.

Reliability and validity

Reliability is concerned with consistency, i.e. the probability of obtaining the same results again. In assessing the reliability of factual questions a number of internal checks can be included. The same question might be asked more than once in a different way. Another form of internal check is to introduce a phoney item, such as a nonexistent brand of puppy food. However, when introducing a phoney item the utmost care must be taken to ensure that it really is a phoney item. Cases have been known where so called phoney items have turned out to be existing products.

Validity is concerned with checking a respondent's account with what actually happened—assuming that there is some other means of verification. A variety of techniques can be used with factual questions. They are known as cross-checks, where a second independent source of information is used. Sometimes records can be used to check on certain points of information, for instance, attendance at a veterinary surgeon. It may also be possible to compare two related respondents such as the co-owners of a puppy. In other studies 'quality checks' are made. This means that some of the respondents who have been interviewed are re-interviewed by a more trained group of interviewers.

Attitudinal questions are more sensitive than factual questions to changes in wording, context, and emphasis. Thus, it becomes impossible to assess reliability if one asks the same question in another form. It is for this reason that sets of questions are used to measure attitudes rather than a single question. The chief difficulty in assessing the validity of attitude questions is the lack of criteria. What is needed is a group of people with no attitude characteristics (criterion group), so that it can be seen whether or not questions discriminate between them. Another form of validation is to compare findings with the results from other studies.

Sampling

Sampling of subjects are selected so as to represent the population under investigation. In order to ensure that selection is representative it is essential that each individual in the population has a fixed and determined chance of selection. This may sound simple but in practice great care has to be taken to ensure that this is so.

Various methods are available for selecting individuals in an unbiased manner according to how the population is listed. The main methods involve either a table of random numbers or a random number generating machine where each individual is given a number and, if their random number is selected, that individual is chosen. (Note: if the individuals are listed in a set order, then only the first member of the sample needs to be selected using random numbers, the rest being selected as every ith number on the list, where i depends on the number in the population (N) and the number in the sample (n), so that $i = N/n$.) Below are listed a selection of various types of sampling techniques all of which enshrine the principle of equality of chance of selection. The type of technique chosen depends on cost and ease of obtaining members of the sample. In general, before choosing a scheme and before selecting a sample, consult a qualified statistician as mistakes at this stage of the research cannot be rectified at a later date.

Simple random sampling, is where in the sampling each individual in the parent population has an equal and constant chance of being selected. In this type of sample no weighting of any sort is necessary. *Stratified sampling* is where the population is first divided into various groups or strata and part of the sample comes from each stratum. *Stratified samples* can be used, for example when individuals of interest to as researcher occur in small numbers in the population, as in the case of a rare disease. Unless an extremely large sample is selected, the number of individuals included with a rare disease is too small for conclusive results to be reached. To overcome this problem, separate random samples are drawn for each of the subsamples, for instance, experimental and control groups. As a result, a higher proportion of minority individuals is selected, although each individual is still selected randomly. Each of the different subgroups is called a *strata*. Provided the researcher knows for each strata the proportion of subjects selected from the population under investigation, it is still possible, by appropriate weighting of the results, to make generalized conclusions about the population. *Cluster sampling* involves selection of random units, such as factories within an industry. All individuals within each of the selected units are then studied. Such an investigation is simpler and cheaper because the investigation is concentrated in a few locations. The technique is less effective than simple random sampling if there are significant differences between the units with regard to the presence of associated factors. For instance, differences between factories to the presence of occupational hazards. In this situation the advantage of a simple random sample is that it is likely to include individuals from all units, and hence shows up better the differences between the units. *Multistage sampling* is where the sample is selected by stages, the sampling unit at each stage being subsampled from the larger units chosen at the previous stage. For example, a sample of factories within the industry may be selected, and then within each factory a random sample selected and stratified by the sorts of jobs employees undertake.

In selecting subjects for a survey, it is important not to exclude subjects because it is difficult to obtain information from them, either because they are not ready volunteers or because information about them is not so readily available, as this would bias the results and make the conclusion of the research invalid. These difficulties may in themselves provide important clues as to the cause of disease but this would need to form part of another study. In all types of sampling the problem of nonresponse and noncooperation can occur and provision for this should be made before starting any survey or experiment by consulting a qualified statistician.

Descriptive surveys

This type of study is concerned with identifying clusters of events according to time, place, and specified characteristics, i.e. when, where, and what. In humans, descriptive surveys usually make use of routinely collected health data, such as that on birth and death certificates and on hospital records. Since this data was not designed for the purpose for which it is now being used, it may be deficient both in quality and completeness. Nevertheless, such data is useful in providing hypotheses as to causation of disease and for initial support of an already formed hypothesis. These results may justify a more elaborate investigation. Since descriptive studies use routine data they are cheaper to carry out than surveys on original respondents.

The main types of time patterns studied in descriptive studies are usually long term and/or cyclical. An example of a long-term trend is the increase in carcinoma of the lung: this trend is similar to those for increased alcohol and tobacco consumption. The descriptive study will be unable to establish whether either factor is associated with increased mortality from carcinoma of the lung, but will identify factors which can be investigated in further studies. One type of cyclical change is that resulting from seasonal variation. Thus gastrointestinal infection is observed to be more common in summer months and a hypothesis can be made that such an infection is affected by bacteria in food which multiply more in warmer temperatures. Again, such an hypothesis could be tested by additional studies. The clustering of events such as disease in different places can also provide useful clues to their cause. Differences between countries point to the influence of ecological, social and cultural factors on the incidence of a disease. Local differences within a country may reflect variations between urban and rural areas. Often diseases are found to cluster within individuals having particular specific characteristics, for example genetic inheritance, age, sex, and ethnic origin. Diseases are also found frequently to cluster according to occupation, socioeconomic group, environment, and culture. It may be just as informative to find that various factors are most commonly found in people who do not have the disease.

Analytic surveys

These are planned investigations designed to define the causes of events more precisely than is possible using descriptive studies alone. Special data collection exercises are carried out with analytic studies and hence they are more time consuming and expensive than descriptive studies. There are two principle type of analytic study, namely the *case control study* and the *cohort study*.

Case control studies

These are retrospective studies in which individual events under study, such as disease, are investigated through direct questioning, and medical and other records with regards to the attributes, experiences, or exposure which are hypothesized as the causes of the disease. This study group is compared with a control group which has the same general characteristics as the study group, except that individuals in the control group do not have the disease under investigation. If possible, each subject in the control group is matched with regard to age, sex, and other relevant factors with each member of the study group. The researcher looks for increased frequency of the suspected causal factors in the study group as compared with the control group. It is the collecting of specific information in both the study and control group that enables the researcher to be more precise as to the possible cause of a particular disease. For instance, the investigator is able to establish through a case control study that although increased consumption of alcohol and tobacco parallels the increased mortality from carcinoma of lung, only tobacco has been shown to be an associated factor. In other words, the researcher will find that the frequency and amount of alcohol consumption is the same in both the study and the control group, but the frequency of tobacco consumption is much higher in the study group.

The case control method does, however, have a number of limitations where:

1. Data to be collected depends on the memories of individuals: these memories may be faulty.

2. The records used for collecting the data have not been constructed for use in the study; they may not always have the exact information required.

3. Although the research can pinpoint more precisely the likely factors associated with a disease, some doubt still remains, very often because the time sequence of events cannot be established. For instance, with carcinoma of the lung the researcher is unable to establish whether chest illness increases susceptibility to carcinomas as a result of smoking, or whether smoking itself brings about the chest illness followed by carcinomas.

4. The starting point for a case control study is one or more individuals with the disease and not the hypothesized cause of the disease. In this case the researcher does not have available representative data as to what percentage of all individuals exposed to a causal factor contract the disease. Thus the researcher is unable directly to establish the risk of contracting the disease as a result of exposure.

Cohort study

The cohort study overcomes the limitation of the case control study as it is a prospective study. On the other hand it is more expensive and time consuming. The main characteristic of a cohort study is that it investigates a group of people before the onset of the disease. In one method of investigation, subjects are selected and followed up systematically over many years. Information is collected as to attributes, experiences, or exposures that are thought to cause a particular disease, and signs of the disease noted. In using this method the cohort provides its own control group. Another means of carrying out cohort study is to select a group of subjects because they have attributes, experiences, or exposures that are believed to be the cause of the diseases under investigation. These subjects are then matched with a control group who have the same characteristics as the experimental group, except exposure to be the factors under investigation.

Analysis of surveys

Descriptive surveys

Descriptive surveys are concerned with formulation and testing of initial hypotheses, through collecting information as to how the disease clusters by time, place, individual, or characteristic. A useful method of analyzing the findings is to use the chi-squared test (see p. 90), setting out the data as shown in Table 12.2.

If clustering of the disease is taking place, the incidence of the disease will be significantly different for the various categories of time, place, or individual. For example, if an environmental hazard is associated with the disease, there will be increased incidence of the disease for places nearest to the hazard. If a category has no influence on the disease the expected (E) value of each cell can be calculated by multiplying each respective column and row total and dividing the product by the total number of observations, for example if the disease was independent of category 1 the expected frequency in the (1+) cell would be

$$E(a) = \frac{n1 \times n+}{N}.$$

Table 12.2 Analysing data using a chi-squared test

Category	Disease		Total
	+	−	
Category 1	a	b	n_1
Category 2	c	d	n_2
Category 3	e	f	n_3
Total	n+	n−	N

where $n_1 = a + b$ $n+ = a + c + e$
       $n_2 = c + d$ $n- = b + d + f$
                          $N = a + b + c + d + e + f$
       $n_3 = e + f$ $= (n+) + (n-)$
                              $= n_1 + n_2 + n_3$

The chi-squared test would then be carried out by using the following formulae:

$$\text{Chi squared} = \sum_i \left[\frac{(A_i - E_i)^2}{E_i} \right]$$

with df = (3–1)·(2–1) = 2

where A = actual frequency in the *i*th cell
E = expected frequency in the *i*th cell
df = degrees of freedom (see p. 92)

The summation being carried out over all cells.

The probability of achieving such a value of chi squared is then found from a table of chi squared. If this probability is less than a previously agreed level, one would tend to conclude that the categories tested are associated with the disease. If the probability is above the previously agreed level one would then tend to conclude that the categories are independent of the disease (see Chapters 10 and 11 for further details).

Analytic survey analysis

Analytical analysis is usually carried out by comparing the incidence of a disease for individuals exposed to the risk factor, against the incidence for those not exposed; this ratio is called *relative risk*. In a cohort study this ratio can be estimated directly since the sample has been stratified according to exposure or nonexposure to the suspected risk factor. In the case control study, however, stratification is by the presence or absence of the disease, and hence direct information is not available as to the incidence of the disease with and without the risk factor being present. Provided the incidence of the disease in the population is small, an approximate value for relative risk can be estimated for a case control study as shown in Table 12.3. This is sometimes called the *odds ratio* because *a/c* and *b/d* are the odds of having the disease, with and without the suspected risk factor. The odds ratio can also be used to estimate relative risk for a descriptive and a cohort survey. Again the estimate is relatively accurate provided the incidence of the disease in the population is small.

Population attributable risk is defined as the difference between the incidence rates in the exposed and nonexposed groups, that is the risk attributable to the factor being investigated. A moderate relative risk applicable to a high proportion of the population would produce more cases of disease than a high relative risk applicable to only a small proportion of the population. Population attributable risk is only estimated where it is considered justifiable to infer causation from an observed association between a suspected risk factor and the disease. Population attributable risk is an important measure in that it indicates the importance of eliminating the

Table 12.3 Approximate value for relative risk of disease for a case control study

		Disease		
		+	−	Total
Suspected risk factor	+	a	c	a + c
	−	b	d	b + d
Total		a + b	c + d	

Approximate value of relative risk (provided incidence of disease in the population is small) = $(a/c)/(b/d) = ad/bc$.

risk factor as a means of preventing the disease. A further measure of attributable risk among the exposed can be estimated as the incidence in the exposed population, less the incidence in the nonexposed population, divided by the incidence in the exposed population. As with any sample statistic the researcher needs to know how good an estimate it is of the corresponding population parameter. Techniques exist for estimating confidence limits (see Chapter 10) for relative risk, population attributable risk, and attributable risk among those exposed. It is also possible to estimate relative risk for a factor which is protective.

Epidemiological studies

Epidemiology is literally the study of epidemics, but, in practice, it is concerned with the natural history of any disease, examining the associated morbidity and mortality in a population. The techniques are particularly useful when looking for long-term effects, such as the influence of environmental factors on the cause and progress of the disease. An epidemiologist has, however, no control of the various risk factors being studied and must be continually on the look-out for new variables which could be influencing the data. Large numbers of a population must be examined and special techniques and terminology have been developed to analyse the data and to obtain meaningful results.

Morbidity comprises primarily the *incidence* and *prevalence* of a disease. The term rate indicates the population change with time, and the risk the probability of occurrence of an event. Incidence rates are the occurrence of new cases within all those still at risk, whereas the incidence risk is the risk of developing the disease over a specified period of time. The relative risk is the ratio of two or more incidence risks. Prevalence is the proportion of disease within a population, i.e. the level of existing disease within the whole population. A prevalence point is the figure obtained for a set moment in time and the prevalence period the figure over a prescribed period. Prevalence and incidence rates are related, since an incident can become a prevalent case once it has occurred and remains so until recovery or death. Prevalence = (incidence) × (*T*), where *T* is the average duration of the disease or, if there is no recovery, the average survival after occurrence of the disease. The measures used in a particular survey depend on the disease. For diseases that have a short non-fatal course, incidence is the appropriate measure. For chronic non-fatal disease, prevalence is often used. For fatal disease, mortality is the usual measure to apply.

Life tables

Mortality figures obtained for the whole population are termed crude mortality figures, and represent the number of deaths at a given time within all those at risk. Comparing survival pattern of communities and countries, however, requires standardization of data, to overcome differences of age, sex, and other factors, such as ethnic origin and the time of collection. This can be achieved by the construction of *life tables*. Life tables are ways of laying out survival data so that the information can be easily and meaningfully examined, and compared with other similarly arranged population data. The tables used for comparison are generally based on national population statistics. In England and Wales for example the Office of Population Census and Surveys, under the direction of the Registrar General, collects and classifies all deaths by age and disease. These figures provide the information from which age-adjusted life tables are made up. Life tables are either of the current or cohort variety, this classification relating to the survey techniques already described.

In *current life tables* the most recently available age-specific mortality rates, such as those from a population census, are used to calculate the expected survival at each age for a hypothetical population. They are based on the assumption that the mortality will continue to follow the pattern of the available data. Current life tables are used for actuarial life-table analysis, such as by insurance companies, figures being used to assess the risk of death at any particular age. This data, however, represents the findings of a cross-sectional study undertaken at one particular moment in time and does not show the changing patterns (secular changes) of mortality figures. Of more use in biomedical research is the *cohort life table* (Fig. 12.3). This is based on data from longitudinal studies of survival patterns starting at a set point (such as birth, commencing a specific occupation, entering a specific environment, contracting a disease or commencing a treatment regime), and then to follow these patterns through time. The data for the construction for a cohort life table may be obtained in a number of ways. These include:

— A series of cross-sectional studies (for example repeated censuses). Thus, figures obtained from a number of the Registrar General's reports can be used to provide a known standard population against which to compare other specified populations.

Fig. 12.3 LIFE TABLE OF A GROUP OF 100 DOGS

1 Interval since start of study years	2 Number alive at start of interval	3 Withdrawn alive during interval	4 Lost to follow up during interval	5 Number of individuals at risk	6 Died during interval	7 Percentage risk of dying during interval	8 % chance of surviving interval (survival rates)	9 Cumulative chance of survival
0	100	0	0	100	0	0	100	100
1	100	1	4	95	6	6.316	93.684	93.684
2	89	2	0	87	2	2.300	97.700	91.529
3	85	0	2	83	0	0.000	100.000	91.529
4	83	3	1	79	1	1.266	98.734	90.371
5	78	0	2	76	0	0.000	100.000	90.371
6	76	0	0	76	2	2.632	97.368	87.992
7	74	1	0	73	1	1.370	98.630	86.786
8	72	0	1	71	3	4.225	95.775	83.120
9	68	2	2	64	5	7.812	92.188	76.626
10	59	0	0	59	3	5.085	94.915	72.730
11	56	1	0	55	7	12.727	87.273	63.474
12	48	1	1	46	11	23.913	76.087	48.295
13	35	0	0	35	20	57.143	42.857	20.698
14	15	0	0	15	10	66.667	33.333	6.899
15	5	0	1	4	3	75.000	25.000	1.725
16	1	0	0	1	1	100	0.000	0
						100		

All withdrawals, looses to follow up and deaths are taken as occurring half way through the interval.
Columns 1, 3, 4, and 6 represent the raw data. Other columns (C) are calculated as follows:

$C2_i = C2_{i-1}(C3_{i-1} + C4_{i-1} + C6_{i-1})$
$C5_i = C2_i(C3_i + C4_i)$

$C7_i = (C6_i \times 100)/ C5_i$
$C8_i = 100 - C7_i$, i.e. the chances of survival to the next interval

$C9_i = (C9_{i-1} \times C8_i) + 100$

Where i represents the period being calculated.

Life expectancy (L_x = average lengths of survival from the start of the study. It is calculated from columns 1 and 9:
$L_x = \Sigma_{i=0} [(C1 + 1/2) \times (C9_i - C9_{i-1})]$

note $\Sigma_{i=0}(C9_i - C9_{i-1}) = 1.000$ in the above table $L_x = 10.56$.

In this table no new animals were added during the course of the study, but analysis does allow for this when required.

— *Retrospective* collection of data (for example from the hospital notes of a group of patients).

— *Prospective* on-going population studies, such as the study of the natural history of vascular disease carried out in the Framingham community in North America. They can also be based on one or more individual case studies, known as case control studies.

Separate cohort life-tables can be constructed for males and females, for different populations, and from other factors such as smoking and different occupations. Subsequent comparisons may be age-linked or independent. Figure 12.3 indicates the typical columns that make up a cohort life table and the various calculations and indices that can be obtained in this form of documentation. The value of these tables is closely related to the accuracy of the information included at the beginning of each interval, since inaccuracies are magnified as the table progresses. The larger the number of subjects involved, the more reliable the results. However, not all subjects need to have been followed through the complete length of the table and the design allows for subjects to be withdrawn or lost to followup, and new ones to be added at any interval. Mortality is the usual end point, but this is not necessarily so and other end points, such as failure of a transplanted organ or amputation of a limb, may be involved.

The total number of deaths is reported in person-years of observation. The mortality rate is the number of deaths divided by the person-years of observation and multiplied by 1000. It is reported as deaths per 1000 person-years. Mortality figures from a life table may be plotted against time as a histogram and confidence intervals added. Equivalent figures from the life table of a known standard population may be plotted on the same histogram for comparison. The ratio of the observed to the expected number of deaths in this comparison is called the standardized mortality ratio. The expected number of deaths denotes the number of deaths if the age- and sex-specific rates were the same for those of the known standard population. The significance of any difference can be calculated by a 2×2 table for each interval.

Summary

1. Surveys observe naturally occurring events without interfering with them.

2. Surveys usually assess large numbers of subjects and provide an overall picture of events occurring in their natural environment, but the researcher is not in control of the variables and is not usually able to examine precise hypotheses.

3. The questionnaire provides a means of surveying large samples. The interview schedule and mailed questionnaire incorporate different techniques and require careful planning and piloting.

4. Random sampling may be simple, stratified, cluster, or by a combination of techniques. To be valid they must all be free from bias and every individual in the population must have a fixed and determined chance of being selected for the sample.

5. Analysis of surveys may be by descriptive or analytical techniques and these may be prospective or retrospective. Descriptive surveys document the time, place, and character of events, analytical surveys relate events to each other.

6. Morbidity and mortality can be documented by life tables, in which information is standardized in a form that allows comparison.

13. Planning and carrying out an experiment

Overview

Experiments differ from surveys in that they involve planned changes with naturally occurring events to assess how they can be modified. Sample sizes are usually much smaller, as their characteristics can be closely defined and, by controlling the environment, variation can be attributed to the planned experimental changes. Precise sampling techniques are again mandatory and the researcher must at all times be on the lookout for unexpected bias. The choice of a research topic may be based on one's reading around the proposed area of study or it may be chosen by a more senior colleague. Once an unanswered question has been identified it is possible to suggest a possible explanation (hypothesis). An experiment is then designed to test this hypothesis. The purpose of designing an experiment is to provide a means of data collection in which sources of error or interference are unbiased. Experimental design is not a means of proving that the chosen explanation is correct, but rather a system by which alternatives are eliminated. The most common sources of error and ways of eliminating them will be outlined in this chapter (see Fig. 13.1 for the stages in experimental design). The example that will be used is the investigation of the effect of a new drug (D) on the lowering of blood pressure, but it could have been the effect of a food product on weight, as in the KPH study or any other unknown relationship. The unanswered question is whether the drug lowers the blood pressure, the hypothesis is that there is such a relationship and the experiment is designed to test whether or not this is so. The drug and the blood pressure are variables and the research problem is the investigation of the relationship between these two variables.

Design and analysis of an experiment

Variables

The factor being deliberately introduced or modified, is known as the independent (explanatory) variable (the properties of which explain some of the variations in the response). The factor being observed is known as the dependent (response) variable (indicating the outcome). The prediction (hypothesis) in this experiment is that the drug lowers the blood pressure of a subject. In the trial one is assessing the effects

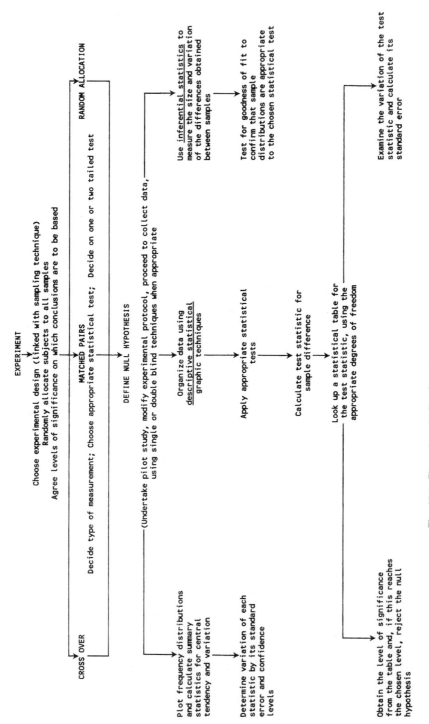

Fig. 13.1 Flow chart indicating the stages in experimental design.

of the new drug on blood pressure and performing an 'hypothesis test' to investigate how likely any effect is to have arisen by chance. The dependent variable may be affected by a number of independent variables other than the drug, and these effects must be neutralized.

Planning

Why design an experiment at all, if one wants to know how a drug affects blood pressure, why not just give it to the subjects and measure the effects? Even if this is done one would still have to make some decisions about the design of the experiment. For example, subjects would have to be selected and a decision made on how much of the drug to administer. If on administering the drug a drop in blood pressure is recorded, this tells one very little. The fall in blood pressure may be a chance occurrence or it may be due to a placebo effect, and any tablet might have the same effect. Moreover, some unrelated event might have taken place between the first and the second measurement of blood pressure or the effect may have depended on the age or sex of the subject. The effect of this type of interference is neutralized by careful planning of the clinical trial and the appropriate introduction of control measures.

Measurement

The apparatus used for measurement, the observer making the recording and even the timing of the measurement are all examples of potential sources of error that need to be dealt with in advance. In studies of the effectiveness of any drug the most important thing is to ensure that the subject takes it. This can be checked by either watching, or by direct administration. Spot blood or urine checks for drug content are similarly a wise precaution. All apparatus should be checked before embarking on the experiment and, if the same observer cannot be constantly used, observer agreement of the measurements taken must be established, for example whether the blood pressure is taken from the right or left arm and when taken in relation to the administration of the drug. In some cases the use of more than one observer might be an advantage, providing observers are allocated randomly to subjects. In this way deliberate observer bias can be spotted and neutralized.

The type of measurement used to record results determines the method of subsequent analysis. Measurement can be classified into three types, these being interval, ordinal, and nominal, in decreasing order of precision. Interval (quantitative or continuous) measurement is measurement as it is usually known, i.e. as on a ruler, this being meaningful subdivisions, consecutive points being at a constant interval. In ordinal measurement (ranking, ordered categories), data points can be placed hierarchially, i.e. they are known to be either smaller or larger than another, but the magnitude of these differences is not known. Nominal measurements classify data into categories, but these categories have no numerical relationship, i.e. it is a qualititive rather than a quantitative measurement. Examples of such categories are colours and if numbers are used they merely act as labels. It is possible to transform higher measurement scales into lower ones, i.e. continuous measurement into ranks and ranks into categories. One technique of measurement occasionally encountered in the clinical field is the *rating scale* which quantifies the severity of such factors as illness or pain; the observer or subject marking their assessment of severity at some point along a line. Such data is usually converted to a ranked form for subsequent analysis. In an experimental design, the method and accuracy (for example the number of significant figures to be recorded) of measurements must be specified. Partial figures must be consistently, raised or lowered, half measures randomized in either direction consistently, and other possible ambiguities anticipated and eliminated. Be aware that some people can suffer from digital blindness or digital preference and exclude such observers. It is also important to try and ensure that the process of measurement does not itself influence the result by creating an artificial environment. In the example of blood pressure, the obvious measure is that of the numerical value of blood pressure, but one could also categorize this into mild, moderate, or severe hypertension, by defining the category boundary according to particular numerical values of blood pressure. This is best done after obtaining numerical values, then different cut-off points can be tried, also it allows for comparison with other workers.

Two concepts demand consideration during measurement, these are the reliability and the validity of a measurement. Reliability refers to the extent to which the same result is obtained on repeated measures of the same phenomenon, for example if the recording device is faulty or not sufficiently precise to measure to the accuracy required, one might obtain a variety of results, reducing the reliability of the measurement. *Validity* refers to the extent to which one is measuring what one sets out to measure. In the case of blood pressure this is rarely a problem, but it becomes important when, for example, one is using a questionnaire (i.e. are the questions 'ambiguous'), or trying to measure behaviour. Note also that the actual measurement of the phenomenon being recorded can also vary due to extraneous circumstances, for example the length of a strip of metal can vary depending on the ambient temperature. Hence to obtain reliable and valid measurements of strips of metal, care must be taken to maintain a constant ambient temperature.

Selection of the subject

The term 'population' in experimental design, does not necessarily refer to the human population, but defines the total number of subjects of a particular type being studied, in this case subjects with a raised blood pressure. One has neither the time nor the resources to study every subject with a raised blood pressure, a group must therefore be selected according to set criteria. These criteria define the population being studied, for example the study may be restricted to a certain age range and exclude subjects who have previously received any hypotensive medication. Ideally, restrictions should be kept to a minimum and the perfect experiment takes subjects selected at random from the whole population. Indeed statistical techniques depend on this random selection of subjects (sample) from a defined population (see Chapter 12, p. 128). Be constantly on the look-out for bias, for example, in the human situation, if the first 20 patients seen in the clinic are all placed in one experimental group and the subsequent 20 patients in a second group, the most severely affected (i.e. those with urgent appointments) may be placed into one group and compared with less severely affected subjects. A particularly interesting source of bias may be the volunteer. These individuals are often highly motivated and suggestible. They are often drawn from a specific social group and may have a particular attitude towards disease. They may also be trained in the subject of the experiment, or may have volunteered because they suspect that medically they have something wrong with them. Similarly, a captive audience of patients or students is certainly not representative of the general population. Any results obtained from tests on this type of sample should only be used for formulating hypotheses and not generalized to the population as a whole.

Number of groups and subjects

The size of a sample will be related to the time and money available for the experiment. However, the larger the number of groups the greater the number of subjects needed to make reliable comparisons. For example, in order to look at different effects according to age, more subjects will be needed than if the age factor is ignored. A useful guide to the number of subjects needed can be obtained from reading the literature on similar problems. Further guidelines can be found in Chapter 11, p. 107.

Control groups

A control group provides a means of reducing experimental error, by allowing one to limit the interpretation of results to a known set of alternatives. The simple situation is when a drug is given and the effects observed. This might be represented as:

M1 D M2

M1 is the original measurement of blood pressure and M2 the second measure with D representing the administration of the drug. As seen, this design limits interpretation of the results. Consider instead the situation:

Group 1 M1 D M2
Group 2 M1 M2

Here two balanced (identical) groups have had the original measurement of blood pressure and a second measurement after a set time but only Group 1 has had the drug. One is now in a better position to attribute a fall in blood pressure in Group 1 to the drug. The design can be further improved by adding a third group of subjects who undergo the same measurements but are given a placebo P:

Group 1 M1 D M2
Group 2 M1 M2
Group 3 M1 P M2

By using this type of design the extent to which the fall in blood pressure measurement is attributable to any or no treatment, rather than to the specific drug being studied, can be established. Comparison could also be made with a drug of known properties administered to Group 2, Group 3 or to a fourth group. Comparison with a known drug serves to overcome the possible ethical problem of withholding drug treatment from subjects in need. Note that the whole rationale of this type of experiment is that the groups must be equivalent. If for instance there is a greater proportion of severe cases in some groups than in others, this invalidates the results. This type of inequivalence can be overcome by randomly assigning subjects to each group or better still by first matching subjects as they are selected (for example according to their level of blood pressure, sex, and/or age and then randomly assigning them to each group. Matching is actually quite a difficult procedure, since some subjects may be very alike on one variable, for example blood pressure, but very different on another, for example age. The more variables that are controlled, the more difficult is the task of subject matching. There is an alternative, however, and this is the situation where each subject is used as his or her own control. This design is always to be preferred in clinical trials, except where long term or carry over effects are suspected (see below).

	Week 1	Week 2
Group 1	M1 D M2	M3 P M4
Group 2	M1 P M2	M3 D M4

In this situation Group 1 receives the drug during the first test and a placebo (or an alternative drug) in the second, while Group 2 receives a placebo in test one and the active drug in test two. In this way variations between the two groups becomes irrelevant since both have experienced each condition. This is called a *crossover design*. It is very commonly used in research, since it is a powerful means of eliminating extraneous variables. It will not work in a situation where the experience of one condition permanently alters the condition of the subject: this is known as the carry-over effect. Neither should it be used in a changing situation, such as postoperative pain. The crossover trial as described above can be further improved. It may be that a human subject can recognize the active drug and the placebo. By making the two treatments equivalent in all respects, for example looks, taste, and smell, one is performing a *blind trial*; in this the subject's expectancy about the effects noted is controlled. A double-blind study is when subjects are allocated to their groups by a third party, so that the observer is unaware of whether the subject is in Group 1 or 2. In this way the observer does not know in what order the subjects receive the drug or placebo until after the analysis of the results; observer expectancy about the outcome is therefore controlled. A triple-blind trial is one in which the person analysing the results is also unaware of the substance administered. The blind trial greatly reduces the amount of bias in the results and therefore adds credence to the final report.

In summary, a population must be defined and subjects randomly allocated to groups for comparison. This comparison may be between groups (controlled by matching of subjects) or within groups (controlled by crossover trials) and the study may or may not be performed blind. These designs reduce the potential error of just administering the drug and measuring the change, but there are a number of further points to consider.

Designed experiments

Controlled experiments are sometimes done on a one factor at a time basis but a far more powerful statistical tool exists, whereby several factors can be tested at the same time. This has the advantage of not only cutting down the number of tests needed to be done, but enables the researcher to examine the interactions between the various independent variables being tested. The theory of the design and analysis of factorial experiments, as they are called, is well written up in the literature and a good statistician will be able to design and analyse an experiment appropriate for the research being undertaken. The purpose of this section is to show briefly how this type of design works and how the results can be tested. Factorial designs and analysis are based on the fact that the total variance (see Chapter 9, p. 79) of a sample drawn from a number of populations can be derived, as an *addition of the variances* of the different populations, and the assignment of the different variances to the different populations is known as the analysis of variance. The variances can be tested by use of the F test (see Chapter 11, p. 115). As an example, suppose when testing the effect of a drug on blood pressure, the sex of the patient is suspected of having an effect on the efficacy of the drug. Separate experiments could be undertaken on males and females and the difference noted. A far better way is to do a two factor experiment where half the males are given the drug and half not, and half the females given the drug and half not. The choice as to who receives the drug and who does not, has to be entirely at random to avoid bias from all the other factors not being controlled.

The experiment is then carried out as follows:

	D_0	D_1	Total
Male	n	n	$2n$
Female	n	n	$2n$
Total	$2n$	$2n$	$4n$

where:

D_0 denotes no drug administered
D_1 denotes administration of the drug
n is the total number of patients in each category.

Note it helps greatly with the analysis if each category (for example male, no drug administered) has the same number of patients. The analysis of the experiment is as follows:

Source of variance	Simplified composition of variance
Drug	$s_D^2 + s_0^2$
Sex	$s_s^2 + s_0^2$
Residual error	s_0^2

Thus one can test the effect of the drug and the sex factor by comparing the amount of variance attributed to the drug s_0^2 and the amount of variance attributed to the sex s_s^2 with the amount of variance arising purely by chance s_0^2. For example one would test:

$$F_D = \frac{s_D^2 + s_0^2}{s_0^2}$$

$$\text{and } F_s = \frac{s_s^2 + s_0^2}{s_0^2}.$$

If F_D is not significant, one would conclude that there is insufficient evidence to say that the drug under test has an effect on blood pressure. If F_D is significant and F_s is not significant, one would conclude that the drug under test is associated with an effect on blood pressure irrespective of sex. If both F_D and F_s are significant, one would conclude that the drug is associated with an effect on blood pressure but that this effect appears to be affected by the sex of the patient. Note the above formulas, both for the composition of variance and the F test, are simplified for illustrative purposes only. This type of analysis and design can be extended further. For example suppose one wished to test whether both age and sex made a difference to the effect of the drug, one could set up an experiment along the lines shown in Table 13.1. The analysis of the experiment would then be carried out based on the following components of variance.

Table 13.1 Experiment to establish if sex and age make a difference to effect of drug

		D_0	D_1	Total
Male	18–25			
	26–40			
	41–60			
	61+			
Female	18–25			
	26–40			
	41–60			
	61+			
	Total			

Source of variance	Simplified components of variance
Drug	$s_D^2 + s_{DS}^2 + s_{DA}^2 + s_0^2$
Sex	$s_S^2 + s_{DS}^2 + s_{SA}^2 + s_0^2$
Age	$s_A^2 + s_{DA}^2 + s_{SA}^2 + s_0^2$
D × S	$s_{DS}^2 + s_0^2$
D × A	$s_{DA}^2 + s_0^2$
A × S	$s_{AS}^2 + s_0^2$
Residual error	s_0^2

Where DxS, DxA, AxS, are the interaction effects of the different factors respectively. Each source of variance for the interactions is then compared to the residual error, using the F test. Should there be any positive interaction effects, the direct effect of any given factor would need to be tested further, by eliminating the effect of the positive interaction. Note that the results of any experiment can only be applied to the range of factors being tested, i.e. in the above example the effect of the drug should not be assumed to work for the under-18s, as these were not included in the test. The two examples of designed experiment given above are only an introduction to the designs that are available and in any given situation it should be possible for a statistician to design a test specifically for the given circumstances. This means that by correct design and analysis of controlled experiments it is possible to isolate the various factors and assess their effects, not only by themselves but also in conjunction with each other.

Multicentre trials

The power of an experiment is very dependent on the number of observations undertaken (p. 105) and it may not be possible to generate sufficient numbers at a single centre to obtain meaningful results. Examples of such difficulties are in the treatment of rare diseases, and conditions where even highly specialized centres have relatively few patients. Positive results may not reach significance and borderline negative results are even less likely to be published and reach a wider audience. The multicentre trial provides a means of obtaining larger numbers and meaningful answers, even when differences are small. They may also allow the examination of various subgroups. Larger numbers are generated more quickly and an answer may be obtained before the work is overtaken by new developments, which could require revision of the protocol. The involvement of a number of centres may highlight institutional, regional, or national differences. However, when they demonstrate uniformity, the results will have a much wider application. Involvement of a number of centres also promotes national and international linkages, and gives a wider exposure to experimental work. Setting up multicentre trials is not without its difficulties. Such studies require a director with sufficient motivation, commitment, and skill to set up, undertake, and complete the project. The director has also to be acceptable to the participants and respected enough to encourage full participation from all the major centres working in the field. The support of a national or international specialist body will facilitate this promotion.

Nevertheless, the choice of director and primary coordinating centre may give rise to personal and political conflict. Furthermore, research is highly competitive and many workers may not be willing to spend a great deal of time and effort on projects for which others will obtain the major credit. The setting up of a skilled team is therefore sensitive but an essential primary step. Agreement must be obtained on the format of the project, the aims clearly defined, standards set, and harmonization obtained on all policies. Experimental design follows one of the forms already discussed, but care has to be taken on the type of randomization and compliance from all centres. The organization of the trial requires a great deal of time, effort, skill, and money from the coordinating centre, under the supervision of the director. Most multicentre trials require a full-time coordinator, adequate office space, and secretarial and clerical help. Data storage and computer time and space must be appropriate, with due consideration given to confidentiality and security. Expert advice must be obtained from statisticians. The filing system must be clearly defined and attention given to the methods of communicating with every centre, with regard to telephone, answerphone, fax, and postal systems. Adequate facilities are needed for photocopying, printing, labelling, and preparing returnable stamped addressed envelopes. The coordinator may well have to visit each centre at the outset of the trial and for regular followup, giving due attention to uniformity of the trial, identifying local differences, checking for compliance, counselling as to the format and tactfully reinforcing all agreed regulations. It is essential that all multi-centre trials have regular feedback, indicating to the participants the status of events, including preliminary results, possibly in the form of newsletters and annual meetings. Although the rewards of multicentre trials can be greater than their locally organized counterparts, the pitfalls are enormous and they do not warrant the necessary expense unless they are undertaken by a fully committed, experienced and enthusiastic team.

Sequential trials

The number of subjects in a controlled trial is usually predetermined and is related to the number of subgroups and the likely outcome. In some situations, however, it may be undesirable to continue a particular form of treatment if it is ineffective. Sequential analysis can provide quick result from a series of trials, when a clear end point exists, perhaps death from a malignant disease. It enables the use of the minimal number of subjects compatible with a significant result and is useful when introducing potentially harmful therapies. Each chart is designed for a specific experiment and the boundaries reflect the chosen level of significance. In Figure 13.2, the results are plotted up or down to the right. If a matched pairs design is being used, tied pairs are discarded from the analysis. The trial is stopped once the score line reaches a boundary. Note: sequential trials have to be specially designed and sampling only terminates according to predetermined rules which are decided by the degree of precision required. Under no circumstances must they be used with ordinary fixed sample methods; for example one must not take an ordi-

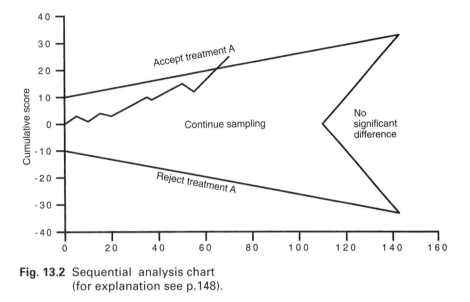

Fig. 13.2 Sequential analysis chart
(for explanation see p.148).

nary sample and test each member one at a time using, say, a t test until a given probability level is reached or not reached.

Pilot studies

At any stage of planning it is possible to run a small pilot study to assess the feasibility of the intended procedure. In the example of blood pressure, there is still the question of dosage. This may be determined by observing the effect of a variety of doses on a group of subjects. Additional studies may be required to determine subject and species variation and the experimental techniques and apparatus must be tested. Similarly in any research involving a questionnaire, a short pilot study is essential to ensure that it is practical and unambiguous to the people using it. A pilot study may also identify unanticipated sources of error. In a blood pressure study for example, the drug side effects may be severe at the proposed dosage, this would need to be investigated more fully before embarking on the trial. All research is time consuming and possibly expensive, so time spent on these initial stages can prevent many difficulties later on. Problems with data collection are often the result of failure at the design stage to anticipate unusual circumstances. A pilot study will help to identify these possibilities. Another reason is to accustom staff with the procedure of the trial. If no amendment is necessary the results from subjects who have been in the pilot study can be used along with those of the main study.

Data recording

The method for recording results must be decided at the start of the definitive experiments. Avoid the urge to record too much information, this can lead to carelessness and lack of enthusiasm by trial participants. Records must be in keeping with the proposed method of analysis and, if a computer is used to store and analyse data, it will save time and effort if the record sheet is planned with this in mind. Precoding, for example Male = 1, Female = 2, makes computer processing easier. Always check that every item has a valid code and there are no gross errors. It is important to code missing values, using some figures outside the range of the measured variable (for example 999). A consistent method of data collection should be used throughout the experiment and it is advisable to have typed pro formas. Always find out from those who complete the form if there are difficulties using it. This can usually be identified during the pilot study stage. The record will usually be handled regularly and a durable sheet is necessary; each record must contain adequate subject identification.

When only one individual is involved with the study his or her characteristic script, abbreviations, and remarks need not necessarily be organized or computed, but if a record is to be interpreted by an independent observer, such as a computer operator or a colleague, these features may require some modification. The layout of a computerized record sheet, must be logical with boxes numbered sequentially when followed down a page. The questions posed should be answerable briefly, while coding information must be precise and printed on the record sheet or in an easily available coding book. The researcher is advised to fill in all information personally, since intermediaries will not necessarily have sufficient knowledge of the subject and ambiguity must be avoided. Some computers are able to scan a record sheet and so avoid a punching operation, but even more care must be taken to fill in such records without alterations, and there must be no open ended question or ones requiring later interpretation.

Data analysis

The availability of computers has made it easy to produce results without ever really studying the raw data. Before starting an analysis, however, one should begin by simply looking at the data, the 'trend' may be quite obvious. Prepare the data in the way that makes comparison simple (Chapter 9). Tables, graphs, and frequency distributions are very important at this first stage and graphing relationships usually improves understanding. The plotting of frequency distributions allow one to check any individual data points which seem extreme or unlikely when compared with the remainder of the data, they also remind one where observations are missing. Although there are acceptable statistical procedures to estimate a value for a missing observation, where possible it is advisable to repeat the observation. Hopefully the number of missing observations will be small and be omitted without greatly affecting the results. Calculators, especially those with statistical functions, have eased the researcher's difficulties of analysis. Great care still need to be taken with regards to positive and negative values and avoid overloading the instrument with many figured digits that are more than the final statistic or significance value require. As a rule of thumb, always work to one decimal place more than will be needed in the answer. Always check the results by repeating calculations, if possible in a different way or having them carried out by a different observer.

Transformation of data

It is sometimes necessary to transform original data into a different form and then to analyse the transformed data. The main reasons for transformation are:

1. To induce normality—many statistical tests require that the data are normally distributed (see p. 103).

2. To arrange that the dispersion of observations is similar across all groups, so that changes in mean are not obscured by greater variability in some groups than in others.

3. To produce simple relationships. For example, by transforming one or both variables an association can sometimes be presented as linear, rather than the more complicated form of the original observations (for example raw scores to logarithmic values).

4. Interpretation is easier if the transformation is physically meaningful (for example the R–R interval of an ECG is the heart rate).

(Note: transformation of data is not always possible and other methods sometimes have to be used in order to ensure valid analysis of the data.) Remember that in order to apply statistical tests all measurements or observations must at some point be described in numerical form, one cannot analyse it until this is the case. All observations can, therefore, be seen as lying along some sort of measuring scale and the intervals along that scale need to be as nearly equal as possible. During the analysis 'variations' will be calculated and if the intervals are uneven the frequency curves will be altered. Transformation may be made on either mathematical or empirical grounds and good statistical textbooks will help one to make this choice. In no circumstances should transformations or other methods be used to distort the data and all conclusions drawn from transformed data must hold for the original data.

Computing results

Some data can be analysed simply with the aid of a calculator. Comparisons using the *t* or chi-squared test (see Chapter 11) for example are very easily analysed in this way. However, most university departments have computer facilities and this will both save time and allow the use of more sophisticated techniques. The staff of computer centres can assist and teach students in the use of apparatus. It is not difficult and the use of computers is an essential part of research training. The first step is to enter the data into the computer in a format which is understood by the statistical package which one intends to use. A package is a collection of computer programs which eliminate the need to do mathematical operations by hand. Many statistical procedures can be performed by these packages.

The form of the results will vary according to the program used. They will look something like the results obtained from analysis by hand, with confidence intervals and significance levels. There will also be a lot of other information, such as the amount of computer time used and any errors in the instructions. Seek advice in picking out the parts of the printout that are directly relevant. At this stage, however, one can begin to see how the results fit the pattern predicted by the experimental hypothesis.

Conclusion

The stages in the design of an experiment can be summarized as shown in Fig. 13.1. The individual case study is also included in this figure and is a special case in research and is often studied retrospectively. It is not an ideal design for generalizing from the results obtained to a larger population and should usually be kept for unique occurrences. It has also been considered under surveys and may prove an important preliminary study to a prospective trial. The identification of an appropriate statistical procedure is an important part of the design and should never be left until after the data collection. The choice of procedure will depend on the method chosen for comparison and the type of measurements used. This in turn will define how data should be collected and recorded. The population, method of sampling, treatment regime, criteria for success, method of measurement, and the required level of significance must always be set before the commencement of the experiment.

The fundamental test of the research method is its reproducibility both by the original researcher and by other workers. Verifiability and replicability imply that data is free from systematic error and personal bias. The examples of error given in this chapter are not exhaustive. There are many more ways in which the blood pressure experiments could be controlled and, although this might make the design and analysis more complicated, computers can help with the complicated arithmetic of more complex statistical techniques. Remember that the interpretation of the result depends on the researcher's knowledge of the field and the confidence with which he or she views the reliability of the data. Even if one treatment is better that another in terms of its desired effect, its complications may be unacceptable and demonstrating that there is no difference in the desired effect of two treatment regimes may be of value if one is less toxic than the other.

Summary

1. Experiments introduce planned changes into naturally occurring events in order to assess how these events are effected and how they can be modified.

2. Measurements may be interval, ordinal, or nominal in decreasing order of precision.

3. The reliability of a measurement indicates its reproducability, its validity indicates whether it is measuring what it sets out to do.

4. The inclusion of control groups, matching between or within groups, factorial designs, and blind trials, reduce experimental error.

5. Specially designed experiments, which enable analysis of variance techniques to be used, are available and are of great value in separating the different effects of different factors. They also enable the researcher to measure the interaction between the different factors.

6. Whenever possible a designed factorial test should be used to test or eliminate extraneous factors. Unless this is done these extraneous factors will either add to the random error, thus reducing the efficiency of any test, or they may become a major source of bias and invalidate the experiment.

7. Pilot studies serve to identify unexpected sources or error and demonstrate the feasibility of the experimental design.

8. Data recording must contain adequate subject identification and be in keeping with the proposed form of analysis.

9. Data analysis can be facilitated by the use of computer techniques but this must always be preceded by the examination of the raw data with descriptive statistical techniques.

14. Computers in research

Overview

The speed at which computers are able to carry out the simple and complex tasks for which they have been programmed make them a desirable research companion. The microchip has reduced the cost and the size of computers, ensuring their widespread availability in the research field. Every researcher should therefore know the basic format of the computer, how to use one, and what to look for when buying their own computer. The terms personal computer and PC are trade marks of IBM, other makes conforming to IBM standards should be termed PC compatible. The other main industrial standard is the Apple Macintosh.

Characteristics and capabilities

Computers may be micro, mini or mainframe, depending on their size and capability. However, advances in technology are tending to blur this separation. In general a micro is a PC, a mini is suitable for a department, and a mainframe computer is capable of handling the simultaneous needs of a large institution. The central processing unit (CPU), program and data memory stores, the input and output systems, and the peripheral attachments are termed hardware. Attachments include keyboards, visual display units (VDU), additional storage units, tape or disc drives, scanners, printers, and modems.

The central processing unit

The CPU is the hub of a computer and in it arithmetic and other logical sequences of operations take place. In the current generation of computers the CPUs are made up of a number of integrated electrical circuits, housed in a silicon chip. IBM chose INTEL to produce the chip for their first personal computer (PC XT) in 1981 and the 8086, the 8088, and later versions have sustained the PC market every since. The later chips were more powerful, being able to deal with a number of bytes (individual pieces of information) at a time and undertake a number of tasks simultaneously. The 80286 chip was used in the IBM PC/AT (advanced technology) computer and for a long time supported a large range of the mid-price computers on the market. The subsequent 386, 486, and the more recent 586 chips are more powerful and the mid-price range of PCs are now supported by the upper range of the 386 or the lower range of 486 chips. The 'clock speed' of a chip is measured in MHz, that of the original PC/XT was 4.7 MHz, that of the subsequent ranges has varied. Common speeds for the 286 are 6–25 MHz, for the 386, 20–33 MHz, and for the 486, 20–66 p MHz. From the user point of view, different speeds affect the computing time. Time is also influenced by the time it takes to retrieve information from the disk and the way in which the video board processes information.

Some of the computer's integrated circuits are programmed by the manufacturer with permanently stored operating instructions and are referred to as the read only memory (ROM). Other circuits, known as random access memory (RAM), are available to the user for entry of other programs and data, and for data processing. The RAM differs from the ROM in that its circuits are cleared of information when the power source of the computer is interrupted. This may be intentional, but power cuts and power surges, and the effects of adjacent heavy machinery may temporarily interfere with CPU function. It is therefore wise to put processed data into storage (back-up) as frequently as possible when running a program. The use of timed back-ups, and roll forwards and backwards is essential if you are on a network. Also to use power surge protectors, these guard against power surges and are available from electrical stores. In the case of power cuts, plugs should be disconnected, as even with the machine switched off, the power surge on reconnection can be enough to damage the hard disk.

Memory

The capacity of the ROM and RAM is measured in bytes. These units are a measure of the number of characters that can be held in a memory at any one time. One byte (b) can store one character. A kilobyte (kb) is 1024 b (this unexpected number reflects that the organization of a computer is based on a binary rather than a decimal system, the number being 2^{10}). A megabyte (Mb) is 1024 (2^{10}) kb. The same units are applied to peripheral stores, such as magnetic tapes and disks. Disks may be floppy, hard, or optical (laser). Floppy disks are made of thin plastic and are coated with magnetic material; they range from 3–8 in. (7.5–20 cm) in diameter. They carry between 100 kb and 2.88 Mb, depending on their diameter and the density of packing. The commonly used 3 1/2 in. (8.75 cm) disk carries 720 kb in its double density form and 1.44 Mb in its double-sided high density version. When buying a new computer, this size of drive is recommended. Hard disks are magnetic coated aluminum and can have a considerably larger capacity, for example a 320 Mb disk is available. Hard disks may be built into a computer: common capacities are 20 and 40 Mb disks, but there is often the potential of replacement with a larger disk. The new generation of optical disks can carry in excess of 14 000 Mb of information, but these require specific disc drives. The various capacities are easier to appreciate if one considers that an A4 sheet of single space typed text requires about 4 kb of storage space. A floppy disk can thus take up to 600 A4 pages, a hard disk approximately 25 000 and an optical disk can take the entire Encyclopedia Britannica. Extra memory may be required to run a number of programs simultaneously, such as printing data while processing other material. Graphics and complex statistical programs may also make heavy demands on memory. Databases can manipulate large amounts of material but this can be held in peripheral stores, only a part being transferred at any one time into the RAM for processing.

Facilities for transfer onto magnetic tape provide a means of storing large quantities of data but tapes are slow to access and when this information is again required it is copied onto disks for further processing. Although more durable and much faster than the floppy disk, a hard disk is more easily damaged, for example by moving the computer when running, from mechanical wear, and if dust comes into contact with it. Information can also be lost by adjacent magnetic fields, power surges, lightening, and inadvertant or malicious clearing of stored material. Multiple switch-ons are more damaging than running time and the computer should be left running unless it is not needed for 6–8 hours or more.

Another malicious source of damage is a computer virus. This is a computer code within a program, capable of replication and spreading to other computers. The damage produced can vary from mild irritation to complete destruction of the contents on a hard disk. The danger is increased when the machine is being used in an institution, or there is a likelihood of coming into contact with other computers, for example, by modem or transferring disks. Consideration should therefore be given to a virus scanner/disinfectant stored on the hard disk. Always scan floppy disks, if they have been on other computers, and all information received by a modem. New viruses are currently 'being released', so anti virus software must be updated. A registered user can have their antivirus software updated either free or at a discount. One should also be aware that viruses can get into printers, if these have a memory, and some have been known to hide in printers and then reinfect a computer after it has been disinfected.

Input systems

The input command systems of computers vary. The commonest form is that of a typewriter-style keyboard, usually with an associated visual display unit (VDU). Whereas such a keyboard is essential for entry of text, when commanding the CPU, additional keys are present to choose the various available tasks. Although secretarial help is usually sought to enter large quantities of text, it is desirable that all research workers should develop typing skills and be able to carry out editing facilities on a word processor. The quest to make computers easier to use, i.e. more user-friendly, has led to the development of a number of alternative and less painful methods of access: 'user friendly' typing courses have also been developed. One group of these systems is known by the acronym WIMP (windows, icons, mouse, pull down menus), although the term graphical user interface (GUI) is becoming more common. In these systems the various functions are placed on the screen as options in text or pictures (icons). The choice can be made with a light pencil, a touch screen, or by pointing with a cursor. The cursor can be positioned with a joystick, with a device known as a mouse, which is moved around on a surface in front of the operator, or by arrow keys or tab keys on the keyboard. WYSIWYG (what you see is what you get) interfaces show the document on the screen exactly as it will be printed out. This makes typing documents, such as reports and questionnaires, much easier. It is found in some Windows and Apple packages. Options are presented as a character-based display in some machines. Menu-driven systems simplify and speed up the choice of function. An input device may read specifically designed cards, be they punched or pencil marked, such as in MCQ examination sheets. Voice-activated programs are under development.

Electrical signals may be fed directly into a computer for storage and/or analysis. They may be generated from another computer, from a storage device or from an external source. In the biomedical field the latter include physiological measurements. Monitoring equipment may contain microprocessors, transforming their measurements into appropriate signals. Another consideration is the need to convert analogue data into the digital requirements of a CPU. Direct transfer of electrical information avoids time and effort, and the potential error of human involvement. On-line analysis provides the rapid availability of physiological results and the possibility of feedback control of a physiological system. In the latter circumstances, consideration has to be given to electrical safety, for example by isolating the subject from the equipment by an optical interface. Such a system must also be designed to recognize and reject artifacts: alarm mechanisms must be built in to prevent inappropriate feedback.

Display

The screen display on most current computers is adjustable. However, the screen size of VDU usually contains half a page of text and this can become very difficult to read if the screen diagonal is less than 8 in. (20 cm): 10 in. (25 cm) or larger screens are more appropriate. Note must be taken of clarity, brightness, contrast, glare, reflectiveness, and the degree of distortion. In colour screens, note the quality of each component and its brightness. Screens should have contrast and brightness controls, enabling these to be set for ambient lighting conditions, and they should not have a highly reflective surface. The screen should have a swivel or tilt mechanism, enabling it to be correctly positioned for the user. Positive image polarity (dark characters on light background) is good if there is a choice, as this provides better readability and legibility, when compared with negative image polarity. The overall illuminence is higher, thereby causing the user's pupils to constrict, leading to a greater depth of focus and reduced accommodative effort. It also means that the display is more compatible with normal office illumination and is less susceptible to glare. Flicker can be higher than for negative image polarity but this is not usually a problem.

The smallest unit that is shown on a screen is a pixel and the larger the number of pixels, the better the definition. The video graphics array (VGA) shows up to 16 colours at a time when the screen is made up of 640 by 480 pixels: the super VGA is the current choice of colour systems. The Hercules monitor/display unit provides a good monochrome system; this has 720 by 348 pixels.

Output systems

Processed material can be examined on a VDU, it may then be stored or the output signal used to drive another device. However, a 'hard copy' is usually obtained through a printer. The directions on when, what and how to print are controlled by the computer, although additional functions may require some memory capability in the printer itself. The speed of printing is related primarily to the printer itself. There are four basic types of printer; a daisy wheel, a dot matrix, a laser, and a bubble/ink jet. A daisy wheel functions as on a typewriter, but is very limited in its number of functions. Only the characters on the wheel can be printed and it differs from the other printers in that it does not provide a proportional font, and it cannot be used to produce complex graphics. The daisy wheel is the slowest of the printers although it produces high quality text; it is not a recommended current purchase. The dot matrix printer produces characters as a pattern of dots produced by pins hitting paper through a carbon ribbon. The laser printer uses electrons to transfer dots onto the paper, the number of dots being of the order of 300–600 per inch (2.5 cm). The fusing temperature required to produce the laser imprint may be in the region of 200 °C. This can be sufficient to damage some acetate overhead projector sheets, sticky labels, envelope gum, pre-existing print on a page, and coloured pigments. This damage may also produce harmful fumes. Appropriate stationary must therefore be purchased. The quality and resolution of print is substantially better with the laser than with the dot matrix printer but in both there is a wide range of quality, closely linked with cost. Additional printer and software features, also influencing quality, include: portrait or landscape format, choice on page size and margins, choice of fonts, print height, width and variety, bold, italic, double stroking; complex graphics, including logos and signatures. Accessories include automatic sheet or line feeds. Colour printing is an expensive but valuable facility. Bubble/ink jet printers give high quality output of 300–600 dots per inch (2.5 cm), similar to the laser printer, but at the same price as a dot matrix printer. They are therefore, a good option if one is on a restricted budget, but still wanting to have a high quality output. Their current disadvantage is that they are slow printers but this is rapidly improving. Bubble/ink jet works by spraying tiny droplets of ink on the paper and therefore high temperatures are not necessary to fix the ink. They can print labels, acetates and have good graphic capabilities. Printers need to be compatible with an associated computer. Usually the correct printer drivers are available, however, if this is not so, a serial/parallel interface board may need to be purchased and fitted.

Software

Additional instructions are loaded into a computer from software packages, usually stored on disks. These may be divided into operating systems and those which provide specific capabilities. The type of the operating system has important implications on subsequent software choice. MS-DOS is the operating system in most PC compatibles and windows sits on top of this, making a computer more user-friendly. Commonly used packages in biomedical research include wordprocessing, graphics, statistical analysis and databases. Other applications include spreadsheets, desk top publishing, programs specific to certain businesses, such as accounting, fax cards, and home computer games.

The computer world is divided between IBM compatible machines and those that are not. Compatibility means that software developed for one machine can also be used on another. Compatibility is also becoming more dependent on the operating systems by which the computer is run. The advantage of IBM compatibility is the availability of a wide range of programs. Non-IBM compatible systems may be superior or more innovative, but the user is unable to benefit from the extensive library of IBM compatible software. This problem is being overcome by the development of emulators which are programs allowing the user to access programs written for different operating systems. All big software houses offer integrated packages either with their full size programs or slightly cut down versions to satisfy individual needs, including word processing, spreadsheets, database, and some graphics and charting facilities. When editing large documents, a fast hard disk and/or clock speed are desirable. Additional graphics packages, for example Harvard Graphics or Lotus Freelance Graphics, are required when composing complex diagrams and preparing slides for projection: they are very useful for the regular presenter.

Wordprocessing

This is almost a universal requirement for the computer user. Many dedicated word processing machines exist and the facility may be a standard fixture in many other machines, this being reflected in their cost. Each system has its own devotees, most provide excellent typing and editing facilities with some graphics. Wordstar was a popular early choice for straight typing and has an excellent spelling check and thesaurus. Wordperfect provides a better visual organization on the screen and handles tables more satisfactorily. Current systems include Microsoft, Word for DOS, Windows, and MAC: other options include integrated packages such as Lotus. Note that some dictionaries are American packages, in the UK look for an English equivalent. Grammar checks are also entering the market.

Statistical packages

Software packages for the PC have often been developed from the programs written initially for large computers. The statistical package for social science (SPSS) is one such example and is an extensive and well-researched system. The statistical analysis system (SAS) is equally powerful but currently, like the SPSS, not very user-friendly; it is widely used in the pharmaceutical industry. In this choice the researcher needs to have a clear indication of the form of analysis required before deciding on the software package. It is worth trying out several packages to see whether their capabilities equate to the likely needs.

Databases and other software

Databases provide a fast means of sorting, manipulating, analyzing, extracting, and presenting data. They have wide scientific application and are of particular importance in patient management and audit. The multiple pieces of information required when documenting diagnosis, details of surgical and medical management, follow-up and outcome, can be linked to each other, and to management information, such as waiting lists, admission policy, bed usage, and patient stay. Database 3 was a well-tried package and has now been replaced by the more comprehensive Database 4. A large number of systems are being assessed with regard to the current interest in medical audit. Paradox is such an example, it being particularly suited to the particular problems of analyzing frequent patient follow-up visits. Foxpro 2 is another much supported package.

The handling of scientific literature provides another example of large amounts of data, in that 6000–7000 scientific articles are produced each day and the scientific database is doubling every 5 1/2 years. Computers form an essential part of data retrieval. On payment of an annual subscription, *Index Medicus* and *Excerpta Medica* databases can be obtained as optical disks, and be searched and retrieved by IBM compatible machines. This software is also available in some non-IBM compatible versions. Bibliographic management software has been developed to create personal databases of references, that can be selectively accessed to produce a bibliography of standard format. Spreadsheets are other programs dealing with numbers, usually in columns and rows. Facilities are present for calculating, analyzing, and sometimes displaying; the programs are designed primarily for simple tasks.

There is an increasing and effective use of computers in education, particularly directed at independent learning, problem solving, simulation techniques, and computer-based examinations. The researcher should consider whether any of these techniques are relevant to the teaching and training of students, and other workers in the field of interest. Further packages may be purpose designed or modified from existing software to carry out specific tasks arising in the research field. Programming is a skilled process and, when unusual tasks are being handled, may take considerable amounts of time. It is advisable to take advice from the local computer unit as to whether a facility for solving a specific problem already exits. A program may well make assumptions, such as normality of data, and these must be checked. If meaningless data is entered the disorder will be magnified and the results meaningless. New programs must initially be checked on small amounts of data.

Expansion

The rate that computer development has progressed over the last decade suggests that upgradability should be of prime concern to a purchaser. The potential to exchange the processor board is available on some computers and this can add power to run new peripherals, such as a laser colour printer, or speed up the use of large software packages. Additional slots to plug in extra RAM and fax cards have already been mentioned. It is advisable to have three or four unused ports for later inclusion of external devices, such as a mouse or modem telephone link. The use of portable units, such as Laplink or Netlite are also cheap and easy options for linking computers.

The commentary so far has assumed that the computer is for individual use. The possible needs of multiple users raise a number of critical questions to be asked of a dealer. Of particular importance is whether the power of the computer is enough to support extra terminals and printers, and how much these will influence the overall response time and speed of all activities, particularly in searching and recording data from large files. It may be wiser to pay for specialist independent advice in these matters. Additional hardware requires extra space and possibly additional furniture. Installation costs may be encountered and the work may disrupt ongoing activities. Care must be taken to avoid loss of data during the additions. Adequate memory, storage, back-up, and archiving facilities must be available, and appropriate means for documentation of all these activities. Links with other computers may be networking by cable or by telephone. Specific problems which arise include:

1. The *style of the operating system*. When a single individual is buying a computer, many features of preference will depend on prior training. The software will not necessarily be equally user-friendly for workers of varying experience: training may be required. The 'help' facilities must be noted, whether these are available on the screen, in a manual or by telephone, and whether the program provides automatic assistance, such as prompts, logical layout, validation manoevures, and warning messages. A group of users may require other facilities such as data retrieval or independent analysis generating reports, and provision of standard and personal letters and labels.

2. *Simultaneous activities*, such as data collection from an analyzer require special locking devices to prevent jamming the computer. Particular attention may be given to tamper-proof keyboards and exclusion of dangerous keys, which could give rise to loss of data or crash the system. It is important to know whether such a loss is restricted to the last entry, a single file or whether it could interfere with a database. Care must be taken to ensure that all material is fully backed-up and careful attention given to auditing, and removing or archiving unwanted data.

3. An *increased number of users* increases the possibility of breech of confidentiality of the material on the PC. Due attention must be given to passwords, at what level of entry they respond and whether these are changed at regular intervals. Certain parts of the file may need to be kept off-line and inaccessible to telephone links or other specified forms of access. Confidentiality must also be considered with respect to maintenance workers and this should be included in maintenance contracts.

Passwords if used should not be dictionary words or names. Ideally they should be a random alpha-numeric (containing at least one digit) string, as these are less likely to be guessed. Many people use their birthday: this would be the first choice for somebody trying to break into the system. One should always change passwords that come installed in a system as these are well known, and provide easy unauthorized access to a confidential system. The problems of viruses have already have referred to.

Display, screen,worker

An awareness of the visual and physical strain produced by continuous work on a display screen has lead a number of countries to formulate laws pertaining to their use. This includes EC Directive 80/270/EC. The latter requires each member state to bring their own laws into line with the proposal. In the UK, the new laws came into into effect at the beginning of 1993. Under these regulations work surfaces must be glare free and spacious enough to allow flexible arrangement of equipment. There should be forearm clearance, with the forearms approximately horizontal. Space must allow the wrists to be rested in front of the keyboard during pauses. There must be enough leg room and clearance to allow postural changes with no obstacles under the desk. Foot rests should be provided if an employee needs one. Chairs must be adjustable in height and back, and with lumbar support. Adequate lighting is required with appropriate contrast and no glare or distractive reflections. A window cover is recommended and distracting noise should be minimized. Screens must provide a stable image, be adjustable for height and angle, readable, and glare and reflection free. Keyboards must be usable, adjustable, detachable, and legible. Software should be appropriate to the task undertaken, adapted to the user, providing feedback on system status and there must be no undisclosed monitor. These regulations will influence future design of computers, chairs, and desks, and demand appropriate attention to be given to work areas.

Choice of a personal microcomputer

Microcomputers present enormous advantages to the researcher. Their relatively low cost makes the purchase of a home computer desirable for the researcher, so that activities can be carried out both at work and at home. This requires transfer of material between the home computer and the usually larger computer of an institution. The transfer is generally by a floppy disk but may be by other means, such as a modem or a portable unit. The uninitiated researcher buying a microcomputer can liken it to buying a car. One is primarily directed by the facilities wanted from it, in terms of power, space and reliability, and the price range. One is also influenced by its looks, handling capability, and other extras one has heard about from friends and salespeople. As with vehicles, there are many publications discussing the virtues of each model and manufacturers provide detailed literature. However, choosing a computer magazine from the vast array in the bookshop is not much easier than buying the computer. The second-hand market is potentially an excellent source of good material but it is very easy to buy a dud. An important difference from buying a vehicle is the existence of a group of computer professionals; it is here that one should start enquiries. Members of the local computing unit will not only advise on equipment but also discuss compatibility with the instrument of the place of work. Consumer association reports in *which* are another good starting place when information searching. They will hopefully enable you to proceed without making a serious mistake. A number of factors must be taken into account, these are considered under compatibility, cost, required functions, and dealers.

Compatibility

A PC may be the prime and only computer being used by the researcher. If, however, tasks are also being undertaken in an institution, the possibility of using the same software at home and at work, needs to be considered. Problems specific to these systems are likely to be known to the computer unit of the institution, and immediate advice can be obtained when sorting them out. It is important however, not to contravene software licensing agreements when reproducing a package on a system, as each package is usually only licensed for one machine and often only one user. It may well be that standardization allows the computer unit to obtain better purchasing deals for members of staff. Buying a machine for research or education purposes through an institution in the UK may avoid the payment of VAT. Dealers may also offer an educational discount and it is worth bargaining to perhaps gain extra software packages in the same price. Standardization on hardware and software is vital for collaborative projects. In such circumstances the researcher may not have the independence of choice, and may be dictated to by a computing department.

Cost

A few examples of various software packages have already been quoted, but these may soon be outdated, as will any costings. The current entry point is the 80386 chip. A comprehensive unit with this chip, with or without a monitor, in the UK, currently costs around £1000. The prices quoted may include a complete unit but a clearly written quotation is necessary: this price may only include a basic nonfunctioning unit. Essential additions that may be needed include an MS-DOS or other operating system, a keyboard, and a VDU. Other possible costs include a printer, a WIMP system, and an extra disk drive. The printer may require an additional card for it to be compatible with the computer. Delivery charges, installation costs, and training have to be considered in the budget. Subsequent costs include software packages, consummables, such as disks, running costs, upgrading, servicing, and insurance. The cost is directly related to the facilities required and the researcher may have to settle for a slower computer, and less programming and storage capabilities, than they would like, with the associated inconvenience of having to carry out certain research procedures only at the place of work. All costs should be calculated as accurately as possible from the outset, in order to plan the budget for the project.

What functions are required?

The chosen microcomputer should be powerful enough to drive the proposed programs at an acceptable speed as judged by computer time, video display time and retrieval time from the disk. Most computers are designed with a specific audience in mind, be they general or specialist, and then provide optimal speed, space, and cost. The 386 range should easily cover the requirements of a single researcher with respect to word processing, statistical package, database, WIMP, laser printer, and if necessary extra graphics. With the potential of expansion, such an instrument is likely to be serviceable for a number of years. Although the power of the 486 seems highly desirable, it is unlikely that individual researchers in most biological sciences require this shopistication. A few exceptions exist, for example a fast mini computer may be required to undertake 3-D molecular modelling.

Software purchased for a microcomputer will usually run on a compatible computer at an institution, but the researcher must check that the reverse is also true. Be on the look out for developments of compatible software that will carry out facilities in your field of interest: further advancements are likely. Once a computer has been purchased it is possible to join clubs and, through telephone links, obtain 'electronic mail' and bulletin boards, which will provide further advice on these matters. Registrants of a user of a particular software will receive announcements about upgrades of products, and may be entitled to free or cheap upgrades. The processing unit, VDU, keyboard, and printer of most computers are not intended for frequent transportation. They may be luggable in a carrying case if absolutely necessary and this weight can be reduced by duplicating keyboard, VDU, and printer at two sites. Smaller computers have been designed to be carried in a briefcase and are useful for travelling. The use of laptops and palmtops is becoming more common, especially with their increased power and memory. Portability, both physical and data, is now the norm. Bubble/ink jet printers of high quality output are also becoming very portable in size, sometimes weighing less than its associated paper store. If the PC is home based there may be other family requirements, these include: bookkeeping, accounting, a dictionary facility, a fax card, and computer games. Although the actual purchase is the end result of the purchasing process, it is only part of an ongoing system life cycle which continues to monitor and upgrade the resources to meet the requirements.

Dealer

It is extremely difficult for anyone to keep up with the changes in technology, let alone implement them. Therefore, it is vital that the 'wave effect' is understood, forms part of the system life cycle, and is merged into the culture of the organization. In reality this means that one purchases every few generations of technology instead of each one, and this is at a pace that the organization is comfortable with politically and financially. The choice of dealer is critical as they must be able to both provide the most appropriate computer and to ensure that it is, and remains, in optimal working order. They should be able to provide a variety of microcomputers and demonstrate the capabilities of each, particularly with respect to handling intended data and obtaining the required performance. Adequate training should also be supplied to the purchaser without excessive charges. The dealer should know the intended developments and expansions in any recommended system. It is essential to chose from a dealer who understands the questions being asked, provides simple, jargon-free, answers and is able to give a balanced opinion. Ensure that the chosen computer and the desired software are available, and determine the likely delivery time: it is frustrating to find problems in this direction following purchase. Find out the track record of the dealer from other customers, with respect to reliability, speed of service, and replacement, and the loan of a compatible computer in the event of failure. Warranties are usually for 1 year and include parts and labour, but check clauses concerning on-site repair and the temporary loan of a computer; these may not be included and are relevant when comparing options. Be careful of cut-price deals as reliability of instruments is essential. Up to 5 years on-site maintenance of a microcomputer should be included in the price by today's market norm. You should no longer have to pay a percentage of the purchase price after 1 year. A computer purchase should be viewed as a capital item over 3–5 years maximum. The alternative to this is to write it off immediately and make the purchase a consumable one. Other options to consider are the rental of a computer and software systems. The latter may be available under the license of an institution but check the expiry date of this license as there may be no reduction in the cost for the use of the program, even when this is only for a short period. Such programs usually contain a 'time bomb' to limit their activity after the expiry. As with a car, the purchaser may have sudden doubts after payment and before arrival of the computer: new models and alternatives are always on the way. However, if advice has been taken, compatibility ensured and expansion potential allowed for, these doubts are unfounded. Once the facility is available and the potential of the instrument realized, all doubts will be resolved and taken over by the pleasures of home computing.

Summary

1. Computers form an integral part of research techniques and the researcher must be conversant with their capabilities.
2. Their common uses in research are: wordprocessing, statistical analysis, organizing large quantities of data, and slide-producing facilities.
3. When choosing a computer, the researcher must decide the functions required and the price range. Advice should then be sought from the local computer department and the instrument bought from a reputable dealer.
4. The researcher has to continue to monitor computer processes to be aware of new developments in the field.

Section C:
Presenting research material

15. Principles of presentation

Overview

Communication of research findings is an integral part of a research programme. It can be manifested in a variety of ways, using the spoken and written word. It is usually commenced by presenting initial experimental findings to departmental meetings and is followed by the presentation of early positive findings to learned societies. Written communications include the publication of papers and possibly a thesis. As work is extended in a specific area, the findings may finish up as monographs or specialist text books. This section considers the various techniques required to present research material in an effective and meaningful way, avoiding possible problems and pitfalls.

The writing of articles and theses, and the presentation of papers and posters to learned societies require just as much training as the other techniques referred to in this book: communicating the findings is as important as undertaking an experiment. Research cannot exist in a vacuum and must not be confined to a laboratory. The researcher has a responsibility to scientific progress to report positive and negative findings and to promote understanding in the field of interest. The researcher also has a responsibility to funding bodies and all co-workers who have given their time and effort to a project. Reports provide the only tangible evidence that any support has been justified. In addition the researcher has the responsibility to himself or herself to gain the satisfaction of completing a project. In some cases this will signal the end of research in a particular field but it provides the confidence to approach future projects in a more informed and efficient manner. The ability to complete and communicate also gains respect from others, often reflected in terms of advancement and promotion in one's field. Such presentations can be assessed for their quality and originality, and indicate background knowledge and training.

What and where to publish depends on how quickly one locates important findings. Initial items of interest are related to new methodology and the preliminary findings: they are usually available after 9–18 months and can be presented to learned societies. The proceedings of these meetings may be published in national journals and, in this way, an abstract of the work will find its way into the world literature. Publications in a specialist journal should represent a substantial contribution to the field. This may well not be until the research project is near completion. It is often at the time of writing up a thesis for a higher degree, when the work is sufficient to produce two or three substantial publications.

Preparing papers makes the researcher examine the project from a different angle. Old literature is reread, perhaps in more detail. It will certainly be accompanied by a deeper knowledge of the field and a new literature search is undertaken.

Research findings are related to this material, conclusions are formulated and ideas clarified, perhaps for the first time. The researcher may have been so involved in undertaking experiments, that the relevance of the findings may not have been fully appreciated.

Reading reports—what to look for

The skills of authorship do not come easily to many researchers. The subsequent chapters go into some detail as to the various forms or presentation. There is a good deal of overlap in written presentations, such as papers, theses, and grant applications and, in turn, with the spoken delivery. This introductory chapter concentrates on what to look for in the writings of other research workers, examining them, as others would examine your own, in an impersonal and unbiased fashion. These techniques will have already been practised in reading early literature and probably involvement in regular journal club meetings. However, at this stage the researcher has considerable insight and knowledge in his or her own field, and is more in a position to ask the necessary questions and provide appropriate answers.

Style. Is the writing simple, direct, easy to understand, and does it follow a logical pattern? Is there any unnecessary material or duplication? Is the article interesting, informative, enjoyable, and worth reading? A satisfactory answer to all these questions indicates a great deal of planning and much rewriting and polishing.

Understanding of the literature. Is the relevant literature included and has it been quoted accurately? If not, does this represent a misunderstanding, misinterpretation, or selective omission? Does the author have enough background knowledge against which to compare the research findings?

Methodology, experimental design and statistical analysis. Does the study have a defined problem? Is the design of the survey or experiment appropriate to investigate the problem? Does the experimental technique allow measurement to the stated level of accuracy? Is the experiment undertaken in a controlled fashion, are the groups equivalent in every respect other than the factor at issue? Are subjects randomly allocated and is there any biased sampling error or other bias? Are the samples truly representative of the population from which they are drawn? Is the appropriate statistical test being applied and are any assumptions, such as normality of the population, justified? Negative answers to these questions reduce the validity of the reported results.

Have all the results been included? Is an original record included and is it calibrated to indicate the accuracy of the technique? Are the tables complete and are missing measurements commented upon? Are the similarities or differences reported, born out by the data or could there be unsuspected findings not accounted for by the level of significance? Could the variation be subject to alternative explanations? Summary statistics, by definition, lose information and the raw data should be available for the reader to verify the accuracy of the calculations.

Opinion of the paper. The reader must decide from the evidence whether the article indicates a substantial and important contribution of original work, and that the writer has shown in-depth knowledge of the field, good judgement, and scientific credibility, substantiating the conclusions drawn. A positive response indicates a skilled piece of research undertaken by a well-trained individual. Irritating features in an article include, repetitive publication, high-profile salesmanship, inaccuracies, omissions, and skating around or fudging the central issues. Of a more serious nature are any departures from accepted ethical codes, misleading reports, and/or downright dishonesty.

Writing reports—pitfalls

Writing up a piece of research as a paper or thesis can become the most difficult part of a research project. The symptoms of pending disaster appear fairly early, with stockpiling of unanalysed data, stacks of unread, unclassified photocopied references, and many piles or disordered sheets of writing and other research material. The end of the research period may arrive with the material still in this state. Additional time is given to the research worker or the material is put aside for holidays or study leave. However, most of each subsequent period is taken up by finding out where everything is and reorganizing it with minimal constructive additional writings. Recognizing the syndrome is easier than rectifying it: it usually indicates lack of adequate supervision. This could be because skilled advice was not available or was not accepted. An argument can be made that if students are not self-motivated nor able to self-assess, they are not ready to undertake a research appointment. It may also be that such students do not have the necessary ability to warrant a research degree. The problem is accentuated, certainly in the UK, by the requirements of most medical graduates intending to follow a hospital career, to obtain a research qualification. To match this need, a large variety of unsatisfactory research projects have to be provided, thus adding to the failure rate. A shorter organized training programme in research techniques would be more appropriate for these individuals, leaving pursuance of independent research to those who demonstrate the appropriate skills. However, in the meantime, the main message in presentation is to start writing in an organized fashion throughout any research period.

Summary

1. Researchers have a responsibility to science, the funding bodies, co-workers, and themselves to complete and communicate research findings.

2. The format of scientific writings follows set patterns. These can be gleaned by exploring the literature, this will also enable the researcher to set their own standards with regards to scientific and ethical excellence.

3. A number of sections, but never the conclusions, of a thesis should be written while still carrying out the experimental work. This facilitates completion of the writing within the scheduled period.

16. Presenting papers and posters

Overview

Once an area of research has been completed it is important for it to be presented to a learned society. These meetings provide a forum for the exchange of ideas between individuals working in the same discipline. The material should be appropriate for the society and represent a positive contribution, based on adequate data. Any dissertation of this kind must not be taken lightly as defects in the research techniques, or the speaker's understanding of the subject, are liable to be highlighted by an authoritative audience. Nevertheless many advantages are to be gained and a student's further research career may depend on meetings of this kind. Moreover, never be overawed by an authoritative audience provided one is sure of ones ground. Many an accepted notion has been changed by arguing with the authorities. This section takes the researcher through the stages of preparing a paper for presentation. It starts with getting the paper accepted and moves on to preparing the text. It then discusses rehearsing the paper and the preparation required on the day of presentation. It ends with guidance on giving the paper and answering questions. Visual aids are considered in Chapter 19.

Getting a paper accepted

The first step towards a presentation is getting the paper accepted: this is usually achieved by submitting an *abstract*. Read the instructions issued by a society, and adhere to these strictly; failure to do so will result in rejection. Keep within the number of words indicated (usually 200–250) and the suggested format. When an abstract form is provided, check the final draft before transferring it into the appropriate space; note also the number of copies requested. The title should include the key words of the paper and be typed in capitals. Write a sentence each, on why the research was undertaken, the methods used, the results obtained, their relation to previous knowledge, and the conclusions. Every sentence must carry weight, as not only does selection depend on it, but it may be published in the proceedings of the society in this form. Phrases such as 'the methods and results will be described' are unacceptable and there is no place for a lengthy introduction, historical data, a literary review, or speculative conclusions. One or more references may be allowed and instructions will state this number, their desired format, and how they are to be noted in the text. One table or figure may be allowed, this will be stated in the instructions to presenters. The instructions may also list accepted abbreviations and units. Divide the text into appropriate paragraphs but limit subheadings where poss- ible to conserve words. The presenter should be the first author and the name of the department should be included, but not the degrees or positions of the contributors. A sponsor's name may be required if no author is a member of the society. The society may require some copies of the abstract to be anonymous. The society may limit an individual to one presentation at any meeting: several papers may be sub- mitted, but if more than one is selected, another member of the team must be substi- tuted as first author or the extra paper withdrawn. When completed, the abstract should be read and approved by all authors, and sent to the society well before the published closing date. Abstracts arriving after a deadline are invariably rejected. An accompanying statement may be required indicating that the work has not previ- ously been presented, published, or submitted for presentation or publication else- where. Papers not accepted for verbal presentation may be offered a place as a poster (or the work may be submitted for a poster). Consideration must be given to whether this form of presentation is suitable, desirable, and feasible (see p. 176).

Preparing the paper

If the paper is accepted, start to prepare the talk immediately, as it will require intensive preparation similar to that of a written communication. Papers delivered to learned societies must contain new findings or new techniques and have to be delivered in a specific time, usually 10–15 minutes. If a presentation is part of a symposium or a lecture, information must be obtained from the organizer with regard to the time allowed, the likely audience and the desired title and content. In these cases the overall plan is similar to a short paper, but the extra time is used to expand on the historical approach to the subject, the details of methodology, and a broader consideration of the implication of the results. If the talk is part of a sym- posium or a conference, the material must be matched to that of other speakers and to the time available. Enquire in advance whether the presentation is to be recorded, whether there will be restrictions on photographing projected slides and whether the proceedings are to be published. These factors may influence your participation and written assurance on these items should be available prior to or conditional on your acceptance to participate. Collect all the material to be presented and arrange it in a similar order to that of a written paper. Introduce the subject, outline the methods, describe the relevant results, and discuss the findings in relation to previ- ous knowledge. Finish by listing the conclusions.

Having assembled the material, it must then be matched to the time available. Initially write out the talk in full in a conversational style and remember that normal conversation is at approximately 120 words per minute (a 10-minute talk equates to approximately three sheets of double-spaced A4 paper). As experience increases it becomes less necessary to write out the talk in full, but the first and the last few sentences must always be written out and memorized. Be aware of the number of new ideas included and introduce each positively, rather than just as an aside. The number of new ideas introduced into a presentation can vary and many rules exist, the better ones lean towards conservatism: stand up, say three things, three times, and sit down; if you cannot remember the flow of ideas in a talk without frequent references to cards it is too complicated; introduce no more than one aspect every 2 minutes, i.e. not more than five in a 10-minute presentation. Such rules are, however, only for guidance and a personal style will soon develop. Finish with a clear summary leaving the audience in no doubt about the intended message. In general the golden rule is (a) tell them what you are going to say, (b) say it, (c) summarize what you have said. Visual aids form an important ingredient of a presentation, they are prepared alongside the spoken material and their function and format are considered in Chapter 19.

Giving a presentation

Rehearsing

The term 'reading' a paper must not be taken literally as many societies discourage reading a paper from notes: such a presentation will in any case 'turn off' even the most enthusiastic audience. The style of the presentation should be in the first person, but not too many 'I's', and must be conversational with variation of form, pitch, tone, and volume. Interest is added by talking to the audience with gesture, movements, and eye contact. The niceties of timing, pauses, and emphasis are only acquired with practice. If a student is not used to lecturing or has a nervous disposition, it is important to rehearse the talk repeatedly. Practice talking to an empty room and listen to a tape recording. Also present the talk to an acquaintance and to a specialist or another worker in the field. It is wise to present the talk, including visual aids, to members of the department a few weeks before the proposed meeting. This timing will allow the format, contents, spelling, and quotations within the visual aids to be checked, and will allow subsequent reorganization, together with additions or omissions to the spoken text. The spoken word must always parallel the messages of the slides being projected. Presenting to a skilled local audience will also provide the likely questions and discussion that will be encountered at the subsequent meeting. Repeated presentation allows a speaker to become fully acquainted with the talk and to establish a firm understanding of all the principles it incorporates. Timing needs particular attention, allow for a 10 per cent increase in length of the presentation due to nerves on the day. Learn key phrases which will direct the line of thought, and can be positively stated even when under stress. While the use of a text for reading the paper is to be decried, the use of prompt cards is perfectly acceptable. These can conveniently be 8×5 in. $(20 \times 12$ cm) file cards on which key phrases or headings can be printed legibly. Visual aids will prompt further key issues, but avoid using them simply as an *aide-mémoire*. Particularly important to remember are the first two and the last two sentences, these must be learned by heart. Do not be overawed or frustrated by the apparent ease with which associates succeed in their presentations: spontaneity is the hallmark of extensive preparation.

The day of the presentation

When the day of the meeting arrives be suitably attired; prior enquiry will indicate the expected dress. Be sure to set out with slides and prompt cards. Allow adequate time to check the arrangements for microphones, pointers, lights, signalling and projection equipment. The microphone may be fixed to a lectern, in which case it should be about 30 cm in front of the chin, there will be marked loss of volume if the presenter continues to talk when looking backwards at a screen. Clip microphones are attached to a tie or dress about 10 cm below the chin, these allow head and shoulder movements towards and away from the audience without loss of volume. Wooden or metal pointers are suitable for small accessible screens, but polychromatic or laser light sources are more commonly encountered. Be careful not to move or damage a screen by contact with a wooden or metal pointer. Lighted pointers may have an attached lead or be battery operated and the beam may be a variety of shapes or colours. Check where the on/off switch is and how heavy the pointer is, whether it can be easily held with one hand for a number of minutes without tremor. Always switch off the light source when not in use and avoid directing the beam at the roof or the audience. The projectionist is usually in control of lighting and will dim the lights to a previously agreed level on request. This level depends on the visual aids. With very dark slides a lectern light may also be required to be turned off, but remember where the switch is when prompt cards are being used. When using bright slides only partly dim the auditorium lights, but turn off the lights over the screen. Most important of all, check the projection facilities. If a film or video is being shown, arrive at least an hour before the published time to ensure that it is set up and tested prior to the arrival of the audience. For 2×2 in. (5×5 cm) slides a rotary drop type of projector is commonly used and it is the responsibility of the speaker to arrive in time to load the cassette provided. Arrival in plenty of time allows the slides to adapt to the temperature of the auditorium: condensation causes a creeping fog across the slide when projected, distracting an audience, at least some of whom will think the slide is about to ignite. Most large meetings provide some form of projector to check the mounted slides before handing the cassette over to the projectionist. Agreement must be reached with the projectionist as to who controls slide advancement and focusing. If this is the speaker's responsibility the facility must be checked prior to the beginning of the session. Check the line of communication with the projectionist, as this may be only through a fixed microphone and communication is lost if a request is not made in the direction of this microphone. There are eight possible ways of inserting a slide into a projector and for most slides only one is correct. On holding a slide up to the light in the upright position, it is standard practice to place a coloured marker disc over the bottom left-hand corner facing you. To project the slide it has to be rotated through 180° so that the marking spot is facing you in the top right-hand corner, the slide being slipped into the slide holder and thence into the projector in this position. If back projection is used, slides are reversed right to left, but not up and down. If a slide is to be repeated, prepare a duplicate and do not expect the projectionist to replace it later in the series. Back-up slides should be carefully numbered so that they are quickly identifiable. Once the slides are mounted the slide holder should be sealed and the presenter's name and the title of the paper attached to it, together with the date, time, and place of presentation. After depositing the slides with the projectionist it is advisable to retire to a quiet area to relax and spend a few minutes thinking over the presentation while looking through the prompt cards. Arrive at the lecture hall in time to meet the chair of the session who will advise on the facilities and on any lighting system used to indicate when there is 1 minute to go and when the full presentation time has been reached. In some presentations the chair may wish to say a few words about the speaker. A good chair will have prepared this ahead of time, but the lecturer should have a few key points ready for a late request.

When it is time to speak, place the prompt cards on the lectern, adopt an upright position and try to look relaxed. Do not put hands in pockets: rest one on the lectern and use the other to hold the pointing device. Do not start until you feel in command of the situation and then speak firmly into the microphone or, in its absence, to the back of the hall. Nerves are more noticeable to the speaker than to the audience. A slow clear voice should be maintained, particular attention being given to names, numbers and formulae. Do not go for extensive walks or talk to the blackboard and avoid repetitive distracting movements and fidgeting. Whenever possible look towards the audience, without engaging the eye of a specific individual. If you dry up refer freely and deliberately to the prompt cards, find the place and resume. A speaker should try to communicate to the audience his or her own knowledge and interest in the subject. Say a few rehearsed and carefully chosen introductory sentences of intent before projecting the first slide, and then have the lights dimmed to an appropriate level. Leave each slide up long enough for those interested to read it completely; this also applies to the last slide. Do not read out the slides but point out features of interest. If a slide is no longer pertinent to the talk have it switched off or insert a blank (opaque or coloured) in the series. Do not be afraid of silence. Finish on a positive note and let it be obvious that the presentation is completed. Over-running time in a scientific meeting is unforgivable.

Questions

Questions provide one of the most important aspects of presentations to learned societies. The chair will decide whether these are taken individually after each paper or after a set of papers. The audience will be interested in learning more about new findings and assessing whether the conclusions drawn are appropriate to the results presented. Many questions can be anticipated and supplementary slides made available, covering aspects of the subject which time did not allow for in the initial presentation. Preliminary presentation of the paper to a home department will probably have identified most areas of interest and uncertainty, but unexpected and awkward questions may still arise. Listen carefully to the question and be sure you understand it. Try to read intelligence into every question, avoiding ridicule or humour, the latter while an enjoyable asset must not be at someone else's expense. If the question has not been heard by some of the audience repeat it and consider summarizing complex multiple questions. Both these procedures allow a little time to think. Answer each question honestly, stating what is known and what is not known, with no evasion of the question. If the answer is 'I don't know' or if an interesting possibility has been raised, say so. If an involved discussion develops with a questioner offer to meet them and complete it at the end of the session. Disagreement should be polite and conclude that different opinions exist. Questioning highlights a speaker's knowledge of the field, together with the amount of thought and effort that has been put into a research project. Handling of intense cross-examination of this nature does much to establish the reputation of a young research worker and can possibly influence future career prospects.

Poster presentations

The success of poster presentations is dependent on considerable planning and good artwork. Acceptance is initially based, not on these qualities, but on an abstract; this follows the same plan as that of a spoken paper, as considered on p. 171. The author may have initially submitted the abstract for a paper rather than a poster. With this in mind, it is essential to balance the acceptance of the offer of presenting a poster with the work required, before agreeing to participate. Specialist societies are usually over-subscribed with abstracts for their annual or biannual general meetings. Many have taken a very positive step to introduce poster sessions to increase the opportunities for members and their associates to present their research work. These societies usually provide excellent facilities for poster display and invite submission of abstracts specifically for posters, or for either verbal or visual presentation. The society may also put aside rooms for chaired discussion of groups of posters based on similar themes, where the author may answer questions from members who have already seen the display. These sessions can provide valuable feedback on the research findings. A prize may be offered for the best poster of the meeting. Organizers of large multidisciplinary and international meetings need to encourage larger audiences and the involvement of as many participants as possible. They will invite many guest lecturers to provide high quality symposia, as well as accepting enough papers to fill all the available lecture theatres throughout the meeting. Once these places have been saturated, they are not in a position to accept any further verbal presentations. However, the organizers still need as large an audience as possible, as registration fees can help to balance the high costs of running such a meeting. One of the alternatives open to them is to accept the remaining submitted abstracts for poster presentations. In this situation the standard required for acceptance may be relatively low and the facilities offered for display may be poor. Discussion may be limited to the author standing at arbitrary times alongside the display to answer questions from chance passers-by.

The above examples represent extremes of a wide range of poster 'sessions', as they have become established in biomedical meetings. The research worker should give full consideration to these factors before submitting an abstract for a poster session, or accepting an offer of a poster presentation based on an abstract originally submitted as a paper. This form of presentation is not necessarily suitable, feasible, or desirable for the available material. The advantages of poster presentations are that any exposure of one's research findings can expand knowledge in the field, it indicates one's interest in the research area, and enables one to meet and have discussions with other workers in this field. The audience can read a poster in their own time and at their own pace, and are not limited to a 5–15 minute presentation at a specific time in a lecture theatre that may have less than ideal facilities. Over the course of a meeting, all interested members of the audience have the opportunity to see the posters; provided the abstracts are published, the posters are numbered, and a plan provided as to their whereabouts. Members of the audience may also come at appointed times to find the author, either alongside the poster or at the set discussion sessions provided. The main disadvantages of the poster compared with the spoken presentation is that a group of experts do not meet together to listen, digest, and criticize the content of the author's work. Other factors considered below are the problems that posters present to the organizers of a meeting and those to the authors in their preparation.

Preparing a poster

The preparation of posters requires specific skills. The text follows the same format as the abstract, containing an initial introduction stating the aims and hypothesis being tested, the methods used, the results obtained, and the discussion or conclusions based on the findings and their relevance to science. The script is relatively short, between 500 and 1200 words. The rest of the space is taken up by illustrations, making the poster as attractive and eye catching as possible, while clearly defining a single message. The starting point is the acceptance of the abstract. The introductory sentences are usually best left to text but the methodology and results lend themselves to illustrative material. A labelled photograph or drawing of the apparatus can highlight new developments, instruments, and techniques. The results may be displayed as pie charts, histograms, or distributions. Graphs can be used to indicate standard deviations or standard errors. It is an ideal opportunity to have photographs of histological or other biological changes. Tables, particularly those including extensive numbers, should be avoided. Much of the discussion may require script but a little imagination will allow the inclusion of illustrations to represent future developments, one to six references may be included in full format.

Once the initial sorting of text and figures has been considered it is essential to know the size of the required poster, its shape and whether the organizers specify specific sizes of type for heading and text. If this information is not available on their literature, the organizers must be contacted immediately to obtain it. White, 1-mm thick flexible card can be bought in 110×80 cm size sheets. When quartered this provides convenient 55×40 cm size pieces which can be fixed to a stand and provide the basis for subsequent stages of preparation of the poster. Four slightly spread sheets fill the basis of the poster space on a 4×4 ft (1.2×1.2 m) stand or two rows of three for a 6×4 ft (1.8×1.2 m) stand. Each sheet also takes two A4 size sheets of paper and two to six photographs. The cards thus provide some idea of the amount of space which has to be covered by the material at subsequent stages or production. Make a scale plan on a large sheet of paper and place numbered blocks representing script, photographs, and illustrations or graphs, across the page. The order of these blocks should follow the sequence of the four sections of the poster but the direction of flow across the page should follow an artistic line, filling the area in a balanced fashion. Try different combinations before settling on a specific design, but avoid crossing card boundaries with any block. Number the cards if the flow is not obvious. Poster headings should be 20–25 mm high and text at least 5 mm, subheadings and key words being 10–15 mm as required. These sizes can easily be read at a metre. Letters should be as bold as possible but capitals should be reserved for headings and important statements. Usually five to eight words will fill a line on each A4 sheet. The labelling on illustrations should be of similar size to the text. The style of the text should follow the recommendations outlined in Chapter 17. The script can be enlarged photographically from normal typescript but, if possible, a composing typewriter should be used and headings prepared by artwork or Letroset. Once the exact size of photographs and artwork have been decided, discuss their preparation with the local illustration department, also discuss the layout of all material, since these workers are skilled artists and designers, and can probably improve the original format. The lack of a skilled department and specialized equipment reduces the quality of presentation and puts the presenter at a marked disadvantage. In these circumstances the emphasis is usually towards additional script and photographs. The preparation of illustrative material is time consuming. Unless it is started at least 6 weeks before the date of the meeting, the author is likely to arrive empty-handed. At an early stage decide whether the backing card should be coloured to improve the contrast of the illustrated material. The text and artwork must be stuck to the card sheets with reliable adhesive and, if the author has to travel any distance to the meeting, it is wise not to build any high projecting models that could be knocked off. The cards provide a useful means of transport as they can be packed on top of each other with an empty sheet on top and tied together to prevent slipping and dislodging of the overlays. Any material passing between cards such as arrows may be carried separately and fixed in position when reconstructing the poster at the meeting. It may be appropriate to produce a three or four page handout for visitors to the stand at the time of the meeting. This can expand on the contents of the poster, extending the number of references and perhaps referring more widely to the author's own work. The author must be present for discussion of the poster at the prescribed times, whether in a specified lecture theatre or alongside the poster. It is often interesting to visit the area at other times to discuss the material with interested readers.

One of the greatest arguments against the time, effort, and expense of poster production is the temporary nature of their use. However, part or all of the display may be retained for at least some months and possibly adorn the walls of a department, serving as a discussion point for visitors and members of the department itself. As a junior member of a large department, one is not uncommonly required to help in running meetings. Experience in presenting papers and posters provides insight into these requirements. The following section considers some of the difficulties that must be tackled in these situations and the standards that should be expected.

Organizing a poster session

The organizer of a meeting should only include poster presentations when adequate facilities are available for such an exhibition. They should also match the number of posters to the available space. If these facilities are available the poster session should be fully advertised, and abstracts invited for posters. Subscribers of abstracts to the paper sessions should be asked to tick an appropriate box as to whether they are willing for their work to be considered for a poster if not accepted for a spoken delivery.

Assessment of abstracts should be by a panel of experts with similar interests to those of the submissions. Selection has to be based on the quality of the abstract, as no indication is available as to the quality of the subsequent artwork: although it is possible that this will be higher when authors have submitted an abstract specifically for the poster session. Assessors should not be tempted to accept more posters than appropriate for the space available, any more than they would chose more spoken presentations than for the time available. Time must be set aside during the meeting for discussion of the posters. These may be chaired sessions within a lecture room but, as these rooms are usually in full demand during the meeting, such sessions tend to be in the lunchtime. The alternative is to indicate the programme times at which authors are stationed alongside their stand to answer questions. This does allow frank discussion between interested parties. It can be very informative for a select few, but large discussion groups moving around the posters are more difficult to organize. It is the responsibility of the organizers to allocate each poster a numbered position and to publish these numbers, along with the abstracts, for the participants. Poster stands are usually 6 × 4 ft (1.8 × 1.2 m) or 4 × 4 ft (1.2 × 1.2 m), the former being 6 ft (1.8 m) long: in both, the vertical span is centred at eye level. The exact size and shape must be communicated to all poster authors. The stands may be wall fixed or free standing, the latter are best if purpose designed, and firmly constructed and stable. To obtain the perspective of a poster the observer needs to stand about a metre away and move a little closer for the smaller print. There should, therefore, be a space of about a metre in front of a stand and facing stands should be at least 2 m apart: 3 m is recommended, to allow groups of observers around the stand without obstructing their fellows. Good lighting must be prepared and this must match the light needed at the time of the meeting (this may be in winter). Additional spotlights may be needed or strip lights over each stand, electrical requirements must be in place in advance of the meeting. It is the responsibility of the organizers to provide the fixtures for poster displays. These will depend on the type of stand, varying from drawing pins and Bluetac to peg boards and various forms of clip. The required number tends to exceed expectations so adequate reserves must be available. Also have stocks of Sellotape, scissors, a variety of glues, a set of coloured narrow and wide felt tip marker pens, pencils, rubbers, a long rule and a stock or white card to help participants in need of emergency repair of their material. The audience must be encouraged to visit the poster display. It should therefore be adequately signposted from all lecture theatres; a further inducement is to have adjacent stations for coffee and tea. Times for meeting the authors for poster sessions should be announced at suitable moments in all lecture theatres.

Overseas presentations

Overseas presentations involving more than one official language present additional problems in preparation. Even more time and thought should be given to the presentation of slides as they may need to be in a different language. If this is required ensure that they are accurately translated as they may be the only part of the lecture that some of the audience will understand. Dual projection allows simultaneous presentation of the same material in two languages but remember the problems that such a technique can present even in a known environment. In verbal presentations, speak slowly and clearly allowing bilingual members of the audience to follow and an interpreter to pass on the information in a meaningful way. Thus, less material is required than for the same time in a home environment. Interpreters may require a script ahead of time to become familiar with the project and to follow during the presentation. Try to ensure that interpreters are familiar with all the technical terms, so that they can provide the correct translation in all the official languages. Delivery in a foreign tongue should generally be avoided unless fluent in the language. This is not to say that the courtesy of a well-rehearsed introductory statement of good wishes in the host tongue should not be included. If an inexperienced interpreter is being used for a foreign presentation the sentences should generally be translated one at a time, and thus less than half the material usually included can be presented in the time allowed.

Chairing a scientific session

Although the new researcher is not the immediate choice as chair of a session, he or she should know the rules, so as to benefit from a good chair, and fill in for inadequacies of the less skilled. The chair of a scientific session plays a specific and important role. Nevertheless the choice is not necessarily related to experience or ability in this field: usually it is based on seniority or specialized knowledge of the topic covered. It may also be a courtesy to a visitor. However, a good chair is necessary for the smooth running of a session. These duties may commence with the organization of a session and the choice of speakers, thus taking on the position of both moderator and chairman. If abstracts are available before the meeting, they should be carefully read, critical facts underlined, and a few comments written down. When abstracts are only available at the meeting, as much time as possible should be allowed to read them.

The chair should turn up well before the start of a session to check the facilities, including microphones for him or herself, speakers and questioners, room lighting and dimming, pointers, slide changers and any coloured lighting system for indicating the time to each speaker. Facilities should be checked over with the projectionist, together with the means of slide collection and available messengers, the appropriate number of chairs and places should be available for discussion panels. By talking to the moderator or coordinator of the session any changes in the programme are noted together with any notices to be given out, these being written down. Checks should be made that each speaker has arrived and to establish that the presenter is the person indicated on the programme. Check the pronunciation of unusual names among the authors or the titles. Remind the presenter of the time allowed for the presentation and questioning, telling them what indications will be given if they are over-running, such as tapping the microphone or using a lighting system: green signifies the allowed time, yellow the last minute, and red overtime. The latter might be flashing and under the chair's control. Talk through the facilities with each presenter and make sure that they are appropriate to the presentation, such as double or overhead projection facilities, blackboard and chalk.

Starting on time is important but can be difficult, particularly at the commencement of a meeting when there may be no audience. Every speaker must get a fair share of the time, however, and delay must be avoided. The chair and speakers must speak into any standing microphone and clipped on microphones must not be covered by clothing. Introduce each speaker by name together with their place of origin and co-authors, provided the list is not too long, and read out the title of the paper. It is the duty of the chairman to provide the optimal environment for each speaker, some of whom will be inexperienced and nervous. The auditorium should be called to order and appropriate level of lighting and focusing requested from the projectionist, if this is inadequate and the speaker has not requested it. Time keeping is one of the most important jobs of the chair. It is not only the inexperienced presenters who go overtime; many seniors do not know when to stop or consider their seniority gives them the right to over-run. Nevertheless no speaker should be allowed to take liberties at the expense of the rest of the programme. Should they not respond to the agreed signals they should be reminded and then asked to come to an end after the current slide. More vigorous intervention is difficult but should always be made in the context of how the overtime is affecting the rest of the session.

In question time the chair should keep an eye on the whole room giving everyone a fair chance and directing a roving microphone as appropriate. Try to pick questioners with a known interest in the topic, but do not let anyone take over or try to deliver a separate paper; make sure to control the verbose participants. If no questions are forthcoming start the ball rolling with some comment or question, possibly based on previous reading of the abstract. The chair must, however, avoid hogging the question time, even if it is his or her own field. Rather they should guide discussion with clear questions and statements. It may be the chair's duty to summarize a session or lead the discussion. Preliminary preparation can produce a series of questions which can be asked at the beginning of a session and re-examined after the papers, examining various aspects of the subject in an orderly fashion. If a speaker does not turn up the decision to bring forward subsequent papers or fill the time with discussion is related to the form of the meeting. In large multidisciplinary meetings with parallel sessions it must be remembered that members of the audience often plan to move around at set times to hear specific papers and topics and times are therefore best left unaltered. International multilingual sessions can be more difficult to chair, requiring more tact. Nevertheless, they should follow the same principles enumerated, with fair apportionment of time to all participants.

Hosting a visiting speaker

Departmental meetings can be greatly stimulated by outside speakers. The young researcher can contribute to discussions on the choice of these visitors and benefit from the wider experience and opinions they provide. They may well be involved in organizing the meeting and entertaining the guest. Guest speakers must be chosen to match the proposed audience with regards to topic, content, and lecturing ability. This choice may be based on personal acquaintance, recommendation or reputation. Unless the speaker is well-known to the host, the initial approach is best by letter and this must include: the proposed date or suggested dates, a suggested topic or field, possible content, and the make up of the audience, the length of the presentation, and the lecture time, the names of any other expected speakers with their topic and any proposed panel discussion, and the details of the lecture hall and projection facilities. A truthful indication is also required of the likely size of the audience, the formality of the occasion, whether refreshments are being provided before and/or after the lecture, if travel or subsistance allowance are being provided and whether there is any lecture fee. This information may encourage or discourage the speaker but must be clearly understood by both parties from the outset of the correspondence. If the speaker accepts, the host should advertise the occasion to its maximal potential and choose a chair who in turn should obtain some background information on the speaker. The host should send a reminder to the speaker two weeks prior to the lecture. This should include travel arrangements, if the speaker is arriving by car, route maps, maps of the local geography of parking, and a temporary parking permit. Details of the lecture theatre should be included and where and when the host or a named deputy will meet them. On the day, the speaker should be met as arranged, allowing enough time to see and check the lecture facilities, set up slides and also to meet a selected few of the audience, possibly over some refreshments and to visit the toilet facilities. At the lecture, the chair should spend a few minutes introducing the speaker, outlining his or her credentials and the reasons for the choice of speaker and topic. The chair should also manage all aspects of the presentation and subsequent questioning (p. 181). On completion, the chair or a delegated member of the audience should deliver a few words of appreciation. During the visit the host should unobtrusively present the speaker with a cheque covering the agreed expenses or indicate when these can be expected. The following day a letter of thanks should be sent by the host to the speaker.

Summary

1. The stages of presenting a paper are getting it accepted, preparing the text and visual aids, rehearsing, getting everything ready on the day, giving the paper, and answering questions.

2. The paper is accepted for presentation on the basis of the abstract submitted. Every sentence of the abstract must be both succinct and contain an important message, the sentences must convey what the researcher sets out to do, why it is important, the main outcomes, and the contribution that the work has made to biomedical knowledge. In preparing the paper be clear as to its purpose and the audience for whom it is intended. Just as in writing a paper, start by constructing a framework on the main sections to be included. Style should be conversational with short sentences which are free of jargon. The paper should convey clear messages, and there should be no more than one new concept for every 1–2 minutes of speech. Write the outline of the text on prompt cards.

3. Rehearsing the talk is essential. This should first be done in an empty room in order to get the timing right as well as to improve on phrasing and emphasis. It is useful to record some of these presentations so as to be able to critically evaluate the performance. Once satisfied, get a sympathetic, but critical colleague to listen. Finally, present the paper to a knowledgeable audience, this will give the investigator a feel for the likely questions, as well as helping to improve the presentation. It is important to include visual aids in the later rehearsals.

4. On the day, arrive early enough to become familiar with the surroundings in which the paper is to be given, to check the acoustics and become competent in the handling of all equipment. If using slides, time needs to be allowed for inserting them correctly into the container. A few minutes in conversation with the person chairing the presentation, sorting our introductory comments and the handling of the session, is valuable use of time. Finally find a few minutes to spend on your own, collecting your thoughts, and psychologically preparing for a good performance.

5. Following all the presentation and rehearsal, enjoy presenting the paper while at the same time be sensitive to the mood and interest of the audience, adapting accordingly, but never at the expense of running over the time allocated.

6. A chair must ensure an optimum environment for all speakers, maintain the publicized time schedule, and facilitate maximum benefit for the audience from the discussion time.

7. A host should ensure that a speaker is fully aware of the terms and conditions of a guest lecture, that as large and as enthusiastic an audience as possible is present, and that the hospitality offered is optimal.

17. Writing papers and reports

Overview

Research findings should be published as soon as they come to a definite conclusion and represent a significant breaking of new ground, even if the results are negative. This chapter takes the researcher through the stages of preparing an article: who should be included as an author, in which journal to publish, and details the preparation of the text. The accompanying tables and illustrations are considered in Chapter 19. Consideration is given to obtaining permission from copyright holders to use material, and guidance included on corresponding with the journal editor and reading proofs, following acceptance of the article for publication.

Authorship

The possibility of writing up a piece of research work should first be discussed with co-workers and senior colleagues. Frank discussion at this stage can also sort out any problems of authorship. Any author should have made a substantial contribution to the work, but remember that a senior person, such as a supervisor, may have formulated the main ideas behind the work, even if a student provided most of the energy. It is important for a student to be well directed in setting out the material for publication and this is more likely if a senior person is closely involved. An established author is also more likely to be accepted by editors. Some journals insist on authors being placed alphabetically and this should also be the case if the work has been equally distributed. First authorship should otherwise go to the prime mover in the research and the last authorship to the senior member of the team. The Vancouver reference system proposes that the order is determined by the authors themselves. Never include anybody as author without obtaining their approval and never allow one's own name to appear in any paper unless fully conversant with the work being presented, and having approved of the version to be published. The standard of any article contributes to both the reputation of a research worker and that of the department where the research was undertaken.

Where to publish

Once a piece of work is complete, decide the form of journal to which it is suited, whether of general or specialist interest. General scientific journals such as *Nature*, and those of general medical interest, such as the *New England Journal of Medicine*, the *Lancet*, or the *British Medical Journal*, have a large distribution and a rapid turnover, but also have a high rejection rate. Specialist journals are more likely to accept articles in their field but suffer from long delays in publication time. The length of article will influence the choice of journal. Extensive reviews are limited to a few journals and most are commissioned or written by established authors in their field. Once a journal has been chosen, become acquainted with its format by reading current issues and the instructions it gives to its authors. The latter are usually included in all, or specific, volumes and can also be obtained from the editorial office. The editor will also require a statement that the work is original and has not been submitted simultaneously to other journals or been accepted for publication elsewhere.

Starting to write

Some authors are able to draft their work on a typewriter, or better still a word-processor, while a few can dictate directly onto a tape recorder. The majority, however, have to prepare their first draft in long-hand. Very few people find it easy to write well, and it is often difficult to know when and where to start. The instructions to authors of the proposed journal will have the required section headings (see below). A possible way of starting is to make notes on separate sheets for each of these headings.

When starting to write, it is advisable to have a working title and to write an abstract answering the questions: why the work was undertaken, what was done, what was found and the relevance of these findings. Once this has been achieved, the research worker should have a clear idea as to the content of the article, and will be able to keep strictly to the point when writing about the work. Use large sheets of paper and leave spaces between the lines for alterations. It is best to concentrate on the content of the article first and then to examine style. From the very beginning, however, try when turning notes into sentences, to write short paragraphs so that they can be easily numbered and rearranged at a later date. Keep the writing simple, clear, and precise using everyday language, avoiding figures of speech and jargon. Do not use long words when short ones will do, or foreign phrases when an English equivalent is available; if it is possible to cut out a word, do so. The text should be intelligible to a nonspecialist as well as to workers in the field. Give preference to writing in the active voice. Check the journal style, most writing is impersonal: on rare occasions personal opinion may be given, but use the third person for reporting what happened. The past tense is best for specific conclusions, but use the present when discussing the relevance of the findings.

Organization of the manuscript

Although scientific journals differ considerably in their 'house style', they tend to follow a similar general pattern. It is worth examining the common headings used in the biomedical field: the title; the abstract and key words (and/or summary); the text—introduction, methods, results and discussion; acknowledgements; and references. Besides the text, tables are used to present findings and illustrations to supplement the text. The preparation of the text is considered first: the preparation of tables and illustration are considered in Chapter 19.

The title page

A working title was suggested as a possible starting point for the writing, but this will usually have to be made more concise for the final version. It should be accurate and informative. It should include the key words of the paper, since many retrieval systems rely on the title for their indexing; do not include abbreviations, jargon or formulae. It is best kept to less than 100 characters, including letters and spaces (approximately 12 words), but a short running title of 40–50 characters may also be acceptable, placed and labelled at the foot of the title page. Also on the title page place the first name, middle initial and last name of all authors with their highest academic qualifications (one or two, as requested), position held and place of work. Indicate which author will be responsible for correspondence and reprints.

The abstract and key words

The abstract should be a concise account for the purpose of the research, the methods, the findings and the conclusions, written in the third person. It must include all the important messages to be conveyed, since this may be the only part of the paper read by many readers. It should not include any material not in the text and should be complete in itself without references or referral to tables and illustrations. Abbreviations should be avoided. The length of the abstract should be less than one-tenth of the paper, this being about 150–250 words for most journal articles. A number of journals require key words or short phrases for indexing purposes; provide three to 10 of these, based where possible on established headings, such as those published by *Index Medicus*. Some retrieval systems provide this complete abstract in a literature search, again emphasizing the need to include all relevant material within the specific wordage. In some journals a summary may be required as well as, or instead of, an abstract. It is placed at the beginning or the end of the article, depending on the house style of the journal. Its length should not exceed one-twentieth of the paper and it should neither be a reworded abstract nor an abbreviation of the whole paper. It is directed at people who have already read the paper and should outline for these the reason the research was undertaken. Emphasize new methods and findings and note conclusions which have been made.

Unlike the abstract, it can refer to the tables and illustrations within the paper. A summary in a foreign language may also be required.

The text

The subdivisions of the text will depend on the chosen journal: introduction, methods, results and discussion are a common arrangement, with subheadings included as necessary. The *introduction* should state the aim of the research, how and why it was carried out, and relate it to similar work, using a few carefully chosen references. State the hypothesis being tested. The introduction should not be an extensive review, two or three paragraphs being usually sufficient.

The *methods* should be of sufficient detail to allow a reader to repeat the experiments. This includes all surgical procedures and anaesthetic techniques. The choice of subjects, exclusion clauses, the variables measured, the form of analysis, and the chosen level of significance, should be defined. If previous publications by the author's group include full details of extensive methodology, such publications are better referenced, and just an outline included on this occasion. State why the method was chosen and define its limits and any assumptions made. Standard techniques may be indicated by a reference, but all modifications of these techniques must be described and methods of statistical and other analysis included. Give full details of control subjects. Specify all drugs and chemicals, including their generic name, dosage, and route of administration. Trade names should generally be avoided, but if included should have a capital letter and, on first mention, should be followed by their generic description. Include in the description all new or unusual apparatus and, where appropriate, the name of its manufacturer. Many journals adhere to SI units, with the possible exception of blood pressure (mm/Hg), but check the instructions to authors. In human studies do not include individual's names, initial or hospital numbers. Indicate that the informed consent of a patient had been obtained and approval given to the project by the departmental ethical committee. In animal studies state the genus, species, race, strain and breed, and where appropriate, the age, sex, weight, source, and methods of housing, handling and feeding. The methodological description should follow a logical, possibly chronological, order and, if it is extensive or complicated, it is better to start with a general outline.

The *results* must be written either chronologically or graded through varying degrees of complexity. The construction of tables and illustrations is considered later, their contents should be referred to, but not repeated, in the text and important measurements should be emphasized. Present the results in as near the original form as possible, where measurements have been summarized, state the extent of variation and the number of observations. When percentages are used for calculation, the actual number of patients/subjects, and the number of observations on which they are based, should be included in the text and the tables. Include all the material that is to be referred to in the discussion, and remember that unexpected and negative results may be as important as expected and positive ones, to future progress.

The *discussion* should follow a logical sequence but not necessarily the same one as the results. This section should not usually exceed half the length of the paper. On reaching each discussion point, state the findings, referring to the result section, together with deductions and their implications. Relate findings to the work of others, being sure to quote original papers and not reviews. Some of the references will have been quoted in the introduction. If the results differ from those of other workers, or unexpected results have been obtained, do not ignore them but try to explain the findings, or state that this has not been possible. Any criticism of other research must be directed at its scientific content and never personally at a author. Throughout the discussion distinguish clearly between fact and supposition and limit the latter to statements that can be tested. Where appropriate, include recommendations and indicate new lines for further study. Always state any assumptions that have been made about any outside factors and conditions.

A *conclusion* is required by some journals and this must not be a repetition of the discussion: it should include a sentence on each important finding of the work, whether positive or negative. It may include other comments on the feasibility of the method, positive or negative results, with their relation to previous knowledge, and the implications on future practice and research.

One or more *appendices* may be added for bulky material which is not essential to the continuity of the text, such as alternative methods, lists of manufacturers, and additional results. Appendices are usually presented and edited with the initial manuscript. They are placed before or after the reference section. On rare occasions, the editor will allow the addition of important information, which has come to light between the time of submission and publication of a paper, as an appendix.

Acknowledgements

These should be brief and courteous, extended to all individuals who have played a substantial role in the research or preparation of the paper. Never acknowledge anyone without their permission since, in so doing, it may imply that they are in agreement with the content of the paper. Acknowledgement may also be made to bodies who have provided funds or facilities for the research to be undertaken.

References

The number of references included depends on the style of the article and the chosen journal. Usually any statement should not be accompanied by more than three references. The accurate documentation of references is the responsibility of the author. Attention to details will ensure that journal reference checking teams will not have to reorganize or question the material. Two main systems are in use for organizing references in the biomedical field. In the name and date system, the surnames of one to three authors, or the first author and *et al.* when more, together with the year of publication are placed in the text, and the bibliography is arranged alphabetically by the surnames of the first authors. In the second system each new reference appearing in the text is numbered chronologically, the number being placed in Arabic numerals in the text, and the author and the year only being included if essential to a sentence. References appearing only in tables and illustrations are given a number appropriate to their position in the text. In the bibliography, the references are placed in numerical order preceded by their number. Even when the chosen journal follows a numerical sequence, use the name and date system for all drafts, also print each reference on a separate sheet containing full details. This allows for addition and removal of reference material without affecting the sequence or order of appearance. If a computerized data bank of references is being used as the source, make sure that the correct reference is identified for subsequent printing. If the journal requires references to be organized in a numerical order, this can be undertaken at the time of the final revision. Systematically look through the text, tables, and illustrations and number the references consecutively on their first appearance. Names and dates can then be crossed out where they have not been incorporated into the text. In the name and date system, ensure that text inclusions are complete, that the required number of authors is quoted and that the appropriate punctuation is used. From the sheet containing the complete reference, compile a reference list in the house style. If in doubt include more information than required and leave the editorial staff to reorganize it. Make sure that the bibliography does not include references not quoted in the text.

When quoting the unpublished work of an individual, add the phrase 'personal communication' after the name in the text but do not add the reference to the bibliography unless the instruction to authors requests it. Any personal communication must be agreed to in writing by the individual quoted. Work accepted for publication can be quoted in the text and the bibliography, 'in press' being placed after the name of the accepting journal in the latter situation. Secondary references should be avoided, but if a reference is only obtainable through a secondary source, quote the primary reference and year of publication in the text and, in the bibliography, the author, year, and 'quoted by' the name and date of the secondary source: also include the full reference of the secondary source separately in the appropriate place in the bibliography. If the references are being used as the reference source, keep them together throughout the time of preparation of the paper but do not have the bibliography typed until the text is nearing completion. When a reference bank is already alphabetically ordered on a wordprocessor, the task of printing out the chosen bibliography for a paper is much simplified.

The Vancouver style of reference layout has been adopted by the large majority of journals world-wide. Journal references start with authors (up to six or three, *et al.* if more) and initials, followed by the title of the paper, title of the journal (in standard abbreviated form), the year, volume and the first and last pages. Books have authors, title, publishers, place of publication, and year. Edited volumes have authors, chapter title, editors, volume title, publisher, place of publication, and year. The style of punctuation can quickly be learned by reference to an easily obtained journal using the Vancouver system, such as the *British Medical Journal*. It is important to follow this style accurately and consistently. The only difference between this style and the recommended style for personal filing is that all authors (i.e. not limited to six) should be included in the latter, together with the source of the reference. Some journals are now requesting a photocopy of the first page of each reference or the title page and chapter page of books. This should be taken into account in one's own system of data storage. Tables and illustrations are prepared at this stage: they are considered separately in Chapter 19.

The typed draft

After the initial long-hand preparation of the manuscript, the next stage is to convert it into a clean typescript for further revision. It is possible that the corrected script is legible enough for a wordprocessor operator or typist to work from, but a rewrite or a dictated version is usually necessary. Indicate that the draft will not be the final version and that minor errors can be indicated rather than retyped. A single copy should be made for each author. All new researchers should learn to type and prepare their own manuscripts on wordprocessors. This saves time and money, and may reduce the number of drafts. Typing should be double spacing with generous margins. During revisions of the typescript at least part of the paper will go through a number of further drafts. It is important to differentiate the different drafts, usually by dating them, but different coloured sheets is an alternative means of coding. When this draft is complete the top copy is retained and each author sent a copy on which to work. Throughout the revisions keep in mind the house style of the proposed journal. The required length of an article is usually about 3000 words and this can be estimated: with double spacing (i.e. three lines per inch), a sheet of A4 contains approximately 350 words. If there is need for a substantial reorganization of the text at this stage, it can be easily achieved on a wordprocessor or, if a typewriter is used, by the cut and paste technique. Many of the comments on rewriting and rearranging scripts are fortunately outdated, with the introduction of wordprocessors with paragraphs shifting facilities. Examine in particular the introduction and the beginning of the discussion; both of these areas are usually too long. Make sure that the latter is not a repeat of the former. The initial title was intended to be a comprehensive directive and can now be streamlined into the final version. Each paper produced by an author should carry a different title, even when covering related topics. Pay careful attention to the organization of headings and subheadings, allowing three to four orders of heading. Scan the paper to check the order of each section and, when near completion, write A, B, or C in the left-hand margin opposite the heading, to denote the degree of emphasis, so that the wordprocessor operator or typist can use the appropriate type and underlining. A possible scheme is to have a central heading of capitals, a side heading of capitals, and side heading with a single capital. Additional headings can be provided by underlining or running the text on in the same line as a heading.

As well as the content, examine the style of the paper. Use simple language avoid jargon, and remove clumsy phrases and unnecessary words. Unfamiliar terms should be defined on their first presentation and terms should be consistent throughout. Reading the text loud, if possible by a person unfamiliar with the subject, will usually indicate whether each verb has a subject, whether pronouns are related to their intended nouns, the presence of noun clusters, split infinitives, and unnecessary adjectives and adverbs. It will also help to add appropriate punctuation and, if written by another person, ensure that what is actually written has the intended meaning, and is not subject to misinterpretation. Hyphens should be limited to situations where they separate repeated vowels and consonants, and when they clarify the meaning of a word.

Abbreviations of a word or words and all acronyms are placed in brackets after the first mention, which is in full; the abbreviation may be used subsequently. As a general rule, full stops are used when the abbreviation is of lower case letters but not for capitals. Proper names should be used for drugs and common trade names added in brackets, with a capital first letter. Subsequent referral may be to either, depending on the emphasis of the article. Most publishing houses will have their own rules on preferred spelling, for example -ise or -ize in verbs, and abbreviations: this can be established by examining a few of their journals or books, other journals specify their choice of dictionary. Some wordprocessors have a spelling check included, but make sure the style is appropriate to the journal or language (for example English or American).

Sentences should generally be under 40 words, but include frequent variation of length. Paragraphs should cover a single topic or part of a topic and generally be less than 125 words, i.e. under half an A4 page. Make sure that the units, their abbreviations and symbols used in the text are those suggested by the chosen journal. When abbreviating isotopes, the atomic number is placed as a superscript prior to the element, and square brackets placed around both when it is being substituted into a compound, for example $[^{14}C]$ glucose. Underline words to be printed in italic script, such as the systemic names of bacteria. In the text, numbers one to nine should be spelt, except when mixed with larger numbers, when they, like these numbers, should be presented as figures. Numerals should also be used for ages, measurements, and statistics. For decimal numbers of less than one, zero should precede the decimal point, and groups of numbers greater than four on either side of the point, should be grouped in threes by a space or a comma. Distinguish equals signs from double bonds, and negative signs from hyphens, by leaving a space on either side of them, except when a negative sign indicates a negative number. When quoting an author in the text, the quotation should be in parenthesis and any words left out indicated by dashes. Any personal comments should be placed in square brackets. If footnotes are to be included in the text, they should be typed between two continuous lines extending above and below them across the page, and placed in the appropriate place in the text rather than at the foot of a page: the publisher will decide their final position when page setting the journal.

Obtaining permission to use material

Check that permission to quote sections of text more than 50 words long, or any illustrations, has been applied for from copyright holders, and also from the authors when they are not the copyright holder. Send two copies of a request letter stating why the material is required and indicate the use to which it will be put. On the end of each letter include a statement of release for the copyright holder to sign and date. By preparing two copies of a request letter, the copyright holder will be able to retain one as a record. Similar consent should be obtained from workers quoted in the text as giving a personal communication. Copies of letters from any ethical committee concerning human and animal research should be submitted to the editor.

The final copy

The final copy should only be typed when the author(s) is(are) satisfied that the text is complete and that a high standard has been achieved. Tell the wordprocessor operator or typist that it is the final version and again discuss the many points of journal style already considered. This copy should be on good quality A4 white paper and typed on a single side using double spacing (or triple if requested) throughout: leave a 2.5 cm (or more if requested) margin all round. Pages should be numbered consecutively in the top right-hand corner and a new page started for each section, these being in the order—title page; abstract and keywords; text; summary; acknowledgement; references; tables; and legends. Ensure that the contents of each section are accurate and complete.

A wordprocessor facilitates a clean top copy of an article. Make sure, however, that the printer matches the machine, with regard to the number of lines per page and the margin size, and that the paper is appropriately placed before printing. Problems can arise with pagination and justification. In the former, standard size page breaks can separate a heading from its associated paragraph and pagination must be checked on the screen before printing. A justified right margin can produce unsatisfactory word breaks or unusual hyphenation. A ragged right margin may be more acceptable. The printer should be the best available in the department; a laser printer provides a higher quality finish than does a dot matrix. On completion, read the whole paper through at least twice. All authors should also read it and at this stage it is appropriate to present it for an opinion to a recognized expert in the field. Any corrections should be made with a soft pencil and placed between the lines and above the error; an additional cross being placed in the adjacent margin. Make sure that all tables, illustrations, and references are accounted for in the text and that they are complete and accurate. Place and encircle the table and figure numbers in the right-hand margin adjacent to where they should be placed in the text.

The editor should be sent the top copy of the typescript and at least one additional copy (two may be requested): together with top copies of all tables and illustrations, including the original art work. Some journals request a floppy disk as well as a hard copy. Keep a copy of everything and send a complete set to each author. Place illustrations in a separate envelope after labelling, and, if they could be damaged by folding, add a sheet of cardboard of an appropriate size. Some journals provide a checklist which has to be photocopied, boxes ticked, and delivered with the article. Keep a photocopy of such a list to hand, even when not requested, as it is disconcerting how often instructions are not followed. The letter to the editor should be formal, requesting consideration of the article for publication. If it is not obvious why that particular journal has been chosen, for example if publishing in a different country or different language, explain the reasons and comment on similar work previously published in the journal. Some journals require, and it is advisable to include, the signatures of all authors of the paper. Ensure that the author responsible for correspondence and reprints has been detailed on the title page, a contact telephone and fax number should be included. Enclose copies of letters concerning ethical approval and permission to reproduce parts of text, tables, or illustrations. A stamped addressed envelope should be included if an acknowledgement of receipt of the article is required.

The editor's reply

There may be a number of weeks delay before a reply is received from the editor. This usually represents the time taken to obtain the opinion of referees. Wait patiently rather than start thinking of submitting the work to another journal. Duplicate publications are a waste of time to editors and readers, and must be avoided. The editor may accept, suggest modifications, or reject the article. If the paper is accepted, consider it a successful outcome to your efforts. The editor may, however, state that the paper will be accepted, or reconsidered, if certain modifications of the paper are made. In this case the author must carefully read these instructions and the reasons given. The editor may be concerned with the size or the style of the article, or expert referees may have commented on some technical factors. An author who has no strong objections to the points made by the editor, would be well-advised to make the alterations, and, in doing so, be assured of a publication. If the author is unhappy about the alterations a letter can be written to the editor. However, the editor and referees are fairly certain to have anticipated such views before making the original decision and it is unlikely that the situation will change. If a shorter article is requested, rephrase the relevant sections rather than just cut out words or sentences. If the modifications requested are extensive and the editor has only offered to reconsider the paper once the appropriate changes have been made, it may be wiser to look on it as a rejection. If the article is rejected the editor will usually give his or her reasons, and these deserve careful perusal rather than heated scorn and indignation. If in doubt, ask the advice of an expert colleague, and if doubt still exists write to ask the editor for further comment. The editor will probably send a more detailed account of the referee's report and may request another expert to review the work. The final decision on publication rests with the editor and it is foolish to persist once his or her opinion is established. Also consider the possibility of wanting to publish in this journal at a future date, and distinguish between courteous enquiry and uncontrolled abuse. Before submitting the work to another journal carefully consider the editor's comments and any others obtained, make appropriate changes. Another editor is unlikely to be influenced favourably by a second-hand manuscript and therefore retype the paper and match it to the style of the new journal.

Instruction	Textual Mark	Marginal Mark
Insert new material	research∧	∧rules.
More space	research∧rules.	#
Insert space between lines	research rules.∕	# or >
Insert punctuation	research rules∧	⊙ ⊙ , ;
Insert hyphen	research∕rules.	/-/
Insert superscript	∕research rules∕.	Ꞌ Ꞌ
Insert subscript	o∧	₂ or ₂
Substitute	research rǿles.	/ü
Delete	research⌐rules.	⌐/
Delete and close up	resbsearch rules.	⌐
Close up	re‿search rules.	‿
Leave as printed	research rules.	stet
Underline	research rules.	underline
Change to italics	research rules.	ital
Change to bold	research rules.	bold
Change to roman	research rules.	rom
Change to lower case	research RULES.	lc
Change to small capitals	research rules.	sc
Change to capitals	research rules.	caps
Transpose	resenach rules.	trans
New paragraph	research rules. [The	np
Run on	research rules.⊃	run on
Move to right	⌐research rules.	
Move to left	⌐research rules.	
Take into next line	research rules. [Ex-	take over
Take back to last line	es research rules.	take back
Invert type	research rules.	invert type
Wrong type (fount)	research rules.	wf
Replace damaged type	research rules.	X
Align	research rules.	= also ‖

Marginal marks are placed opposite the corresponding line of the correction. Divide more than three corrections between margins, placed from left to right in the same order as in the text.

Fig. 17.1 Proof correction marks.

Proofs

After acceptance of a paper, the next stage is the arrival of the proofs, usually in galley form. Attend to them rapidly and return them within a few days. At this stage an author is not permitted to alter the text substantially, although important additions may be allowed as an addendum. Restyled phrases probably correspond to the journal house style, and will be retained even if changed. Proof-reading is a strict discipline and requires meticulous care. Remember that an author's reputation as well as that of the journal will be judged by the final presentation. Checking the proof, with a second person reading the original, is a reliable way of picking up missed phrases or sentences. If this is not possible, read slowly or aloud. Again mark the appropriate position in the text for tables and illustrations by writing in the adjacent right hand margin, and ringing the instruction. Correction of the proofs should be clear and unambiguous. Figure 17.1 indicates the textual and marginal correction marks which should be used by authors to ensure accuracy of subsequent editing. When in doubt, write out marginal instructions in full. All marginal instructions not to be included in the text should be ringed.

Check the numbering and labelling of all tables and figures and the text references. The bibliography is usually checked by an expert and if this is stated to be so, do not attempt to restyle any references, rather note the changes in your copy. Photographic proofs will be presented as half-tone copies and the quality of these reproductions does not represent the likely appearance in print, therefore, accept inconsistency of contrast, but carefully check all letters and symbols. With the proofs will be a request concerning reprints; some may be provided free of charge. It is advisable to limit oneself to this number rather than sustain a large bill. Although publications in a journal with a wide circulation will generate requests for reprints in excess of this figure, regrettably the majority of these requests will be indiscriminate and sent by an efficient secretary or as part of a literature search. Therefore limit distribution (and expenses) to friends, acquaintances, those known to be interested in the subject, and those who may have limited access to the journal or inadequate copying facilities.

Summary

1. The stages in preparing an article are agreeing on authorship, deciding where to publish, preparing text, tables and illustrations, getting permission to use copyright material, corresponding with the editor and, if successful, reading the proofs.

2. The common headings used for journals in the biomedical field are: title; abstract and key words (and/or summary); the text—introduction, method, results and discussion; acknowledgements; and references. Tables are used for setting out findings, and illustrations are used to supplement the text.

3. Once the decision has been made about where to publish the article, it is important to study the target journal closely, becoming very familiar with its format, so that the article to be written can be modelled on it. Examine carefully the instructions the journal gives to authors and note such characteristics as, the number of tables included for every 1000 words of text.

4. Starting with the abstract helps the researcher to focus on why the work was undertaken, what was done, what was found, and the relevance of the findings. Having this clearly and concisely in mind will help the researcher to keep to the point when writing the full article. Since many readers will only refer to the abstract, it is important that this is written well and includes all the important messages to be conveyed. The researcher should come back to the abstract after completing the article, refining it and modifying it as necessary.

5. A useful way of progressing with an article is to take it section by section. Begin by making notes on what to include in the section, and then turn these into sentences and paragraphs. Every day language should be used, avoiding figures of speech and jargon. The aim is for a lay person of average intelligence to understand the text.

6. Text tables and illustrations need to be carefully checked by all the authors. With the initial draft, concentrate on getting the content right and, when satisfied with this, progress to modifying the style of the paper so that it is clear and concise. Check too at this stage that the format of the paper meets with the requirements of the journal. Finally, painstakingly, ensure that words are spelt correctly, the grammar is correct, and all references and cross references are accurate.

18. Writing a thesis

Overview

A thesis comprises the documentation of a number of years work and is the only written evidence which is available to the examiners as to the calibre of the research undertaken: it must therefore do justice to the work involved. The thesis is an integral part of a research programme and writing is a continuous process throughout this period. Target dates for completion of each section must be laid down at the commencement of the research. Writing a thesis requires skill and stamina as evidenced by the 50 per cent of candidates in some fields who fail to submit a thesis within 5 years of registration of its title. Submission in itself, however, does not equate to a successful outcome. There are accepted formats with regard to size, style, and content. This chapter considers the main sections of a thesis, their relative size, and what examiners are looking for in each section and in the thesis as a whole.

Regulations and registration

As pointed out in previous chapters, it is important to make the decision to present the research as a thesis as early as possible in the work. Certain degrees require a set number of years of registration and regulations vary in the time allowed for retrospective registration. Read the regulations relating to the submission of any thesis very carefully: establish whether the necessary preliminary qualifications have been obtained or will be obtained by the time of completion of the thesis. Look for directions on the type of work which is suitable for the proposed degree. Note the layout required for the written presentation, and examine copies of successful theses in the university library. The regulations for candidates who have obtained their primary degree in the same university may differ from those from outside, as may regulations for part-time research workers. If there is any doubt, these matters should be discussed with the university registrar.

The proposed title should be discussed with a supervisor or a recognized teacher of the university. Most application forms require the name of a supervisor or a person conversant with the work. The application requires the proposed title for the thesis, this should be related to an area of research rather than a specific phenomenon, in case the latter is less rewarding. Careful consideration must be given to the title since radical changes at a later date are not favoured by any university, although a subtitle can be conveniently added later. A candidate is not permitted to submit a thesis which has previously been awarded a degree at another institution.

Where there is any overlap, this should be indicated on the entry form and in the thesis itself.

Format

The ease and style of writing varies substantially with different individuals and is considered on p. 186. Much of the thesis is written during the course of the research, but the final bringing together of these parts, and the discussion, is carried out in the last 3–6 months of the research project. The overall size of a thesis is between 200 and 400 pages but check all regulations and examine successful theses in the university library. By this time a candidate is fully conversant with the field, and will have presented much of this data for journal articles and in presentations to learned societies. As each section is completed, pass it out to a supervisor; it is part of the supervisor's responsibility to monitor progress and to provide rapid feedback on progress and future requirements. When sections of the thesis cover areas in which the supervisor is not an expert, consideration should be given to obtaining advice from other sources.

Opening pages

The title page should state the title which has been accepted and approved by the university, the degree for which the thesis is being submitted, and the full name of the applicant. A subtitle may be added to that originally submitted to the university to detail the topic. An acknowledgement page allows the author to extend thanks to various people who have supported the work. The first section is usually the abstract. This should be the most carefully written section of the whole work, indicating briefly (500–1200 words) the stages of the work from its conception: the identification of a problem, the proposed solution, the method of study, the findings, the relevance of the work to scientific knowledge and the conclusion. The section is usually redrafted many times. Some universities ask for a summary rather than an abstract, either at the beginning or the end. The distinction drawn between an abstract and summary when writing a paper (p. 187) is less clear cut in a thesis. When a summary is requested, rather than an abstract, it is recommended that the candidate include it at the beginning, covering the points considered under an abstract. The contents are usually incorporated at this point: plan it during the preparation of each section, including each heading and subheading; the pagination is included after the final typing has been completed.

Literature review

The review of the literature takes up approximately a quarter of a thesis and most of it can be completed during the first half of the allotted research period. It must be comprehensive, covering all the literature related to the area of the study. Relevant papers must be studied in depth, the account being critical rather than purely descriptive. This section will draw on the information collected throughout the study and will include the carefully prepared sentence and quotations already referred to (p. 23). It should cover knowledge of the field to the current time and consider any misconceptions which have arisen. The review forms the basis for comparison with the author's results when writing the discussion. In a rapidly developing field, it can be impossible to keep up with the current literature in an exhaustive fashion, and the writer must be realistic and decide when to call a halt to adding further material.

Materials and methods

The introduction to the materials and methods states the hypothesis being tested, the techniques used, the control methods included and the pilot studies undertaken. The method of analysis and statistics used should be appropriate to the hypothesis and the experimental design. The section as a whole is written during the period of data collection and, with the results, make up approximately half of the thesis. The materials, subjects, and methods section should be comprehensive. The thesis may be the main reference to the investigation and the information included should not leave a reader in any doubt as to the exact steps taken. The work of others should be quoted, indicating if and where it is at variance with the techniques used in the study. Specify all the apparatus used and from where it was obtained; give any operative surgical details. Case histories, where relevant, may be given in full and, if extensive, included as an appendix. Discuss the choice and limitations of the experimental design and define the methods of analysis. State the genus, species, race, strain, and breed of any animal model and, where appropriate, the age, sex, weight, source, and methods of housing, handling, and feeding. In humans appropriate information from this list is included. Give full details of controls and discuss any ethical problems; where appropriate, indicate that the informed consent of any subject has been obtained. Individual names, initials or hospital numbers should not be included but subjects should be identifiable throughout the thesis by an appropriate labelling system.

Include illustrations and photographs where they are applicable but written permission is required from a human subject if an illustration is identifiable. Photographs of animal experiments should be discussed with the supervisor and possibly the Home Office Inspector. Subdivide the section, where this adds clarity, and include this in the contents list.

Results

The results section must be in full and the data must be well-organized, using tables and graphs whenever applicable. Photographs may be necessary but require more preparation (Chapter 19). The layout should be meaningful and consistent and understandable to both the expert and nonexpert in the field. A large number of tables of additional, but not directly related, material may be added as an appendix, either at the end of this section or before the bibliography. It may be helpful to summarize the findings at the end of each subsection of the results. The trends and values reaching the pre-set levels of significance are stated.

Discussion

The discussion should make up at least one-quarter of the thesis. This section should start by recapitulating the problem and relate it to the previous knowledge as presented in the review of the literature. The results are then considered in the light of previous knowledge, taking each fact separately and relating it to previous ideas, indicating its general and specific interest and its originality. Once the results have been related to previous knowledge the author is at liberty to draw any tenable conclusions. In a thesis it is permissable to theorize more than elsewhere, but be sure to distinguish between comments and facts. In completing the discussion also speculate as to the future, but do not leave unanswered questions of the kind an examiner might consider should have been investigated. Where appropriate, include recommendations and indicate lines for future study. Particularly indicate criticism of the research undertaken, stating its limitations and indicate alternative approaches that could have been followed.

Conclusions

Conclusions should be brief, and are best listed. Clearly define new methodology, unique findings, and findings at variance with previous reports and established or commonly held views. It should state how the findings supported or challenged the original hypothesis, what further work is needed and the direction it should take. At the end of this section, when required by the university, include a statement of the *claim to originality* of the thesis as a contribution to science and, in particular, to the field of study. This position may also be used to indicate any conjoint work and any overlap with material presented by the candidate or co-workers for a degree in the same or another university or institution.

Bibliography

The bibliography must include each reference in full (p. 190). If these details have been properly filed during the research it should be possible to take an alphabetical list directly from a wordprocessor or a series of file cards. In the text, authors should be listed in full on their first appearance (unless otherwise stated by university instructions) and subsequently should be abbreviated to one or two authors or, in the case of more than two authors, by the first author followed by et al., and the year of publication. If the authors names are included as part of a sentence, the year is placed in brackets after the names. Reference to personal communications and unpublished work should only be placed in the text.

Printing

Most theses require A4 paper, typed in double spacing with wide margins. Three copies including the top copy are usually required and the author is expected to have a copy for personal use at an oral examination: this may also be bound. Expert secretarial help is advisable at this stage, although the preparation of a thesis provides an excellent opportunity for the research worker to learn to type and become conversant with a wordprocessor. On completing the draft, check the university regulations again, as to the layout, the binding, and the number of copies required. The secretary should receive the complete draft together with a copy of the university instructions. Decide what means of reproduction is to be used, this will usually be a top copy printed from a wordprocessor, with photocopies, but may be a typed copy and carbon copies. Once the manuscript is complete the page number should be added to the contents list. The pages are numbered consecutively from the title page through to the end of the bibliography, including tables and bibliographic sheets or mounts. In addition, figures and tables should have separate numbers and separate indices. The required number of copies must now be taken for binding, university regulations should be checked as to whether reprints of personal published articles on the same topic need to be bound into the thesis or placed in a back pocket. Each university has recommended book binders who can prepare the volume in appropriately coloured art-vellum or cloth, with the year, title, degree, and the author's name printed on it in gold. If presented in December it is usual to date the thesis for the following year.

The oral

At least 2 months elapse after submitting a thesis before further action needs to be taken. This is due to the time taken to appoint examiners and for them to study the work. A decision may be taken on the thesis without oral examination but it is usual to be invited to meet the examiners, they are usually two or three in number, one of which may be the supervisor. Before an oral, put aside 3 or 4 days to reread the work, since some time will have elapsed from the time of writing. Make a list of any errors and take this errata sheet to the viva. Also become acquainted with any further developments in the field. If the examiners are known, be fully aware of their field of interest and where this overlaps that of the thesis. Discuss the viva fully with the supervisor close to the date and anticipate likely questions, such as the strengths and weaknesses of the study, and future research required in the field. The oral can be used to discuss subjects which, although not included in the thesis, the examiners think relevant to the field.

If the thesis is accepted, a copy will be placed in the university library and it may be quoted as a publication. When writing subsequent articles relating to the contents of the thesis, completely rephrase it in the form described under writing a paper. If the thesis is rejected, establish the reason for this as soon as possible. This will be easier if the supervisor is one of the examiners, as he or she will then know the reasons and, as rejection reflects partly on the calibre of the supervision, will want to improve the situation. In the absence of a supervisor write to the university registrar to enquire on the reasons for rejection. Examiners' reports are confidential but if they have suggested resubmission within a certain time, they will indicate the improvement in the work which they require and the university will often release an edited part of the report. If it is not possible to establish the reasons for rejection from the university ask another expert for an opinion. Whatever the course, it is vital to maintain an interest in the field until resubmission or it has been established that the work is unsuitable for the proposed degree. Careful attention to the various aspects of this text should prevent the latter outcome.

Examiners' assessment

It is helpful for a candidate to consider how examiners assess the thesis. Examiners are usually experts in the chosen field and, even if they are not, are experienced research workers, aware of the necessary qualities of good research, and of its difficulties and pitfalls. The number of examiners, and whether the supervisor is one of them, is dependent on the university policy for the proposed degree. When reading a thesis, an examiner will start with the choice of topic, as outline in the title and subtitle. This choice (p. 14) is of prime concern: it must incorporate a degree of originality and be relevant to the field. The examiner must be satisfied that it is of sufficient interest, originality, and importance to warrant a research project. The abstract will be read next and probably more than once in order to obtain an overview of the problem, its investigation, the outcome, the conclusions, and the inferences drawn. The subsequent order of reading depends on the individual's experience, preference, and knowledge of the field. A well-constructed contents list allows the examiner to find the way through the various sections. The conclusion is often read next in order to reinforce this overview. More detailed background information on the subject is obtained from the review and then begins a careful assessment of the methods and results sections and a full appraisal of the discussion. The review must indicate that the candidate is fully conversant with the field of study, has included all pertinent references, quoted all authorities accurately, and provided a balanced account, indicating insight and understanding of the subject. Failure to quote recognized authorities or current (even if unpublished) ideas count against the candidate. Personal communications will indicate that the candidate has communicated with other active workers in the field. These may include one or more of the examiners, although this would not have been known at the time. The hypothesis tested must be clearly defined and the action plan, methodology, experimental design, and method of analysis must be appropriate to the problem being studied, indicating a clear understanding of the subject and ensuring that all critical experiments have been undertaken. The candidate must have completed sufficient experimentation to justify or refute the proposed hypothesis. Emphasis is given to the measures introduced to control error. Positive or negative results are equally acceptable but they must be set out in full and missing readings explained: any hint of fabrication of any result will lead to failure of the thesis.

The discussion receives particular attention from an examiner. Findings must be considered in the light of previous knowledge and arguments followed logically from their conception through to their completion, with justification of the chosen approach. The contribution of the research to scientific knowledge must be stated and discussed. Alternative explanations must be included and placed in perspective, and all questions should have been asked and answered leaving no loose ends. The influence of the findings on current knowledge and future research should be considered in depth. At the end of this assessment, an examiner must be satisfied that these various factors have been successfully completed and the total amount of work involved equates to that of the chosen degree. Combined work and team involvement raise some problems and the candidate can expect further questions on these matters in the oral examination. The examiner must be satisfied that the personal responsibilities and contributions of the candidate are substantial.

Although a thesis is examined primarily on the quality of the research project, the examiners also have a responsibility to ensure that it is well-written and produced in the style required by the university. The universal availability of word-processors means that there should be minimal editorial errors and the bibliography should be laid out in an approved style, and should be complete, matching the text. An examiner usually checks key references, particularly when examining outside his or her prime field of interest. Illustrations should be of high quality (Chapter 19), and the captions of illustrations and tables must be well-annotated and edited, the whole thesis being worthy of publication in the university library.

If no oral examination is required, the examiners will communicate with each other by telephone or in writing, in order to reach their decision. This will not necessarily be unanimous as opinions can differ. However, before finally accepting or rejecting a thesis, examiners usually request an oral examination. In a preliminary discussion, before the candidate joins them, the examiners consider the strengths and weaknesses of the thesis and a question plan is set up in order to clarify these views. In the subsequent oral, ambiguous statements will be clarified, errors corrected, and controversial statements challenged. It provides considerable insight into the candidate's depth of knowledge and personal involvement. The final outcome is based on an overall judgement of the thesis talking into account all the factors listed above. The responsibility of the examiners is to the university, and not to the candidate, to retain the appropriate standards and safeguard quality. The candidate's aim should, therefore, be to satisfy the examiners on all the points mentioned.

Summary

1. Read the university regulations and follow them closely; register for the proposed degree as soon as possible, and in the format directed.

2. Plan and set out in diary form a programme for writing the thesis. Much of the literary review and methodology can be completed early in the research programme and most sections drafted during its middle third. At least 3 months is allowed at the end of the programme to complete and submit a thesis.

3. A thesis is examined on its literary style and quality of editing as well as its experimental content.

4. The title must be registered with the university at the beginning of the research project. Subsequent changes may be difficult, so a short general title is submitted: a more detailed subtitle may be added at a later date.

5. The abstract is the most precisely and carefully written section; each sentence should carry a distinct message. Indicate the problem being studied, the proposed solution, the method of study, the findings, and the conclusions.

6. A contents list is compiled as writing progresses and subsections added as necessary.

7. Make files for each section of the thesis and use different coloured paper to identify early, mid, or final drafts.

8. Writing the literature review starts with information gathering. A detailed organization is required for cataloguing references, reprints, photocopies, and all writings. Classify and retain all bits of information.

9. The review indicates the past and present status of the research field, and forms the basis with which to compare and discuss the research results.

10. The materials and methods section must be comprehensive: this may be the only reference to the techniques used. The information should be such as to allow the reader to repeat each stage of the investigation.

11. The results should include all data. If a large number of tables are included these may be placed separately as an appendix.

12. The discussion relates the results to the research hypothesis and the earlier findings by other researchers considered in the literature review section.

13. The conclusions should be clearly defined, listing items in chronological order.

14. Some universities request a statement on the claim to originality of the work. This is primarily concerned with the contribution of the thesis to the scientific field. This may also be a place to state the contribution of the candidate to any combined work.

15. The bibliography should present the references in the format decreed by the university.

16. The thesis should be set out, printed, and bound in accordance to the rules of the university.

17. Before the oral, the candidate must reread every word of the thesis and be conversant with all further developments in the field since the time of

submission of the thesis. Make a note of any editorial or factual errors which have been subsequently found in the thesis.

18. When writing subsequent articles redraft the material. Do not just reproduce chunks of the thesis, since the style of these two forms of writing are different: the thesis requires in-depth description, presentation, and discussion, while a paper requires concise information on the findings.

19. Illustrating the written and spoken word

Overview

Illustrative material is an integral part of all written and verbal presentations. It must be closely linked to the presentation and consideration given to its format and content early in the preparation. Illustrations may take longer to produce than text and the following paragraphs set out the rules that must be followed in order to obtain a balanced presentation on schedule.

Illustrating the written word

Illustrations can be divided into diagrams and photographs. Diagrams include line or tone drawings, charts, graphs, and histograms. Although computer graphics have markedly facilitated the production of good quality diagrams, such as charts and graphs, for the majority of illustrations a considerable amount of time and effort is required from both the author and the artist or photographer. They should therefore be kept to a minimum and included only after careful consideration as to how they will supplement the text. This rule is less stringently applied to theses than other publications, since there is space for full illustration of all apparatus and techniques assessed and used. Well-produced charts clarify the presentation of data; line diagrams can replace a difficult description; while photographs can demonstrate the quality of the record of a measurement, unique apparatus, and unusual events. Illustrations should be understandable, independent of the text, and provide a separate unit for referral. Wherever possible, in the final publication, they should be on the same page(s) as the text to which they refer.

Diagrams and graphs

Discuss diagrams with professional illustrators early in the preparation of an article, and make preliminary sketches clear and accurate. Provide the illustrator with guidelines on the required format, including any instructions from a chosen journal. Charts, graphs, and histograms should be drawn on good quality paper with black drawing ink to provide a good contrast. Diagrams should be double the eventual size so that minor irregularities disappear on reduction. Lines, letters, and symbols should be thick enough to match this reduction. If large drawings are made the work should be checked through a reducing lens to demonstrate the eventual line thickness, capital letters should be at least 1.5 mm in height. Freehand or standard typed lettering are unsatisfactory and should be replaced by stencils, laser printers, composing typewriters, or Letraset. Some journals request a tracing paper overlay indicating alphabetical and numerical additions, these are then added at the time of printing. The overlays must accurately line up on the drawing (or photograph) by adding a few guide lines. Graphs should be included in addition to tables when interesting trends are present. All graphs must have a zero baseline and both axes should have units clearly marked and labelled at appropriate intervals; add only enough intervals to encompass the curves shown, thus avoiding empty spaces. Histograms may communicate trends better than curves but bar charts should be used for noncontinuous measurements. Words should be written in lower case and placed lengthwise along both the horizontal and vertical axes. No more than four curves should be included on any one graph and the line broken for any symbols used to plot the points, and when they cross each other. The symbols used to plot the points should be unique to each curve, but consistent in related graphs. Symbols and abbreviations should be based on a journals's house style when the material is being presented to a specific publisher. The spelling of units and abbreviations should be identical in the text and illustrations. Where means are being presented, standard deviations or standard errors should also be included, together with the number of observations.

Photography

Photographs should only be submitted when they clearly demonstrate unique situations and the focusing and contrast are sharp enough to obtain a satisfactory reproduction. Most journals request glossy unmounted originals. A suitable size is 7×4 in. (17.5×10 cm) and it should not be greater than 10×8 in. (25×20 cm). Although a photograph can be turned into a full page of a thesis, it is usually more convenient to type the figure number and caption, together with the page number for the thesis on a blank sheet and to dry-mount the photograph on this page. Mounting is left to a late stage in preparation, since such pages can not be easily modified. Photomicrographs should have a scale added and this, like any letters and symbols, must be of sufficient size to allow reduction and be of sufficient contrast to be easily seen. Original records must be calibrated. Where appropriate also include a diagram to indicate the areas of the photograph to be reproduced and any additional labelling. Most journals do not accept coloured photographs, those that do may request the author to pay some or all of the costs of reproduction. In the case of human subjects, identity should be effectively masked if this does not interfere with the purpose of the photograph. In any case the written consent of the patient or volunteer should be sent to the editor. Photographs of animals should only be submitted after consultation with a Home Office Inspector. Cropping should be indicated on a tracing paper overlay, or an attached diagram or photocopy. The photograph itself should not be marked. If details in the photograph extend to its margin, and 'Do not crop' to the instructions on the back of the photograph. Completed diagrams and photographs should be numbered consecutively, but independent of any tables, using Arabic numerals. When submitted to a journal they should be labelled on their back or on an overlay, using a soft pencil or a sticky pretyped label, indicating the top of the illustration, the author's name, the title of the article, and the figure number. Under no circumstances should a biro or hard pencil be used on original artwork or on any surface of a photograph. Felt tip pen markings may be inadvertently transferred to the front of a photograph and be impossible to remove without damaging the print. Paper clips should never be applied directly to the front of a photograph. Legends submitted to a publisher should be typed on a separate sheet, consecutively and correctly numbered. They should describe the diagram or photograph, but be short (not more than 50 words) and supplement rather than duplicate the text. Magnification and staining techniques should be added to the legend of photomicrographs and all symbols and abbreviation defined. Ensure that diagrams and photographs relate to the text at all stages of their preparation. When a series of diagrams relate to the same topic, symbols and abbreviations should be consistent throughout. If any diagram or photograph has previously been published, written permission must be obtained from the individual holding the copyright and suitable acknowledgement made.

Tables

The tables in a paper or thesis usually represent the basic research findings and they should be designed to convey this message clearly. They provide a concise way of presenting material particularly of a numerical form. The information they include should be complete and independent of the text and need not be repeated in the latter, which they should supplement rather than duplicate. Study recent copies of a chosen journal and note the usual number of tables included for every 1000 words of text. Examine their size, shape, and organization, together with the symbols and the letters or numbers that are used for sub- or superscript.

Titles should be brief and placed at the top of each table. Tables should be typed in double spacing and each placed on a separate sheet of paper, independent of the text. When a number of tables cover the same area they should be uniform, numbered consecutively in Arabic or Roman numerals, depending on the journal style. The column headings should be short or abbreviated and include the units of measurement of the figures they contain. Although a table is intended to portray maximum information in minimal space, do not overcrowd them. If necessary divide a table into two but, if it extends onto a second sheet, repeat all column headings precisely.

Numbers in columns shouid be in line with decimal points directly beneath one another. Related measurements should be placed in adjacent columns: vertical and horizontal lines to separate columns and rows are unnecessary. Define all sub- and superscripts and all abbreviations in a footnote included in the table and not on a separate sheet, but use footnotes as sparingly as possible. Abbreviations common to a number of tables can be defined on the first appearance and referred back to in the legends on the later tables. Statistical details should be included, together with the number of observations from which they are derived. All numbers in tables should be rounded as much as possible without loss of essential information. Spurious accuracy confuses.

It is advisable to prepare tables at an early stage, as it is helpful to have them nearby when preparing the text. This also ensures consistency between tables and text; this must be maintained at all stages in the preparation. The final appearance should be compatible with the 50 per cent reduction on printing. The publisher should receive the original typescript rather than a photocopy. If a table is conveying only a little information, consider carefully whether this information would be better included in the text. The desired position in the text of tables and illustration should be marked in the margin with the corresponding number and identifications.

Illustrating the spoken word

Visual aids

Visual aids comprise slides, overhead transparencies, black- and whiteboards, flip charts, film, video, and computer graphics. Technological advances may well improve these commonly used aids, and their potential should be fully assessed. Visual aids should be carried in hand luggage when travelling by air, as they are less likely to be damaged and a talk must still go ahead even if other luggage is lost or delayed.

During the preparation of the script for a spoken presentation consider the type of visual aids which will be needed. Visual aids are such a prominent part of present day talks and lectures that audiences are conditioned to require them. What is equally true, however, is that badly chosen or ill-prepared visual aids can mar an otherwise good performance. The visual material must be pertinent to the script and supplement rather than duplicate it. Preparing visual aids requires planning and takes time for art and photographic departments to complete them. Even when preparing the material oneself, it is imperative to plan well in advance in order to avoid going to a meeting empty handed or with unchecked material. The current preference of visual aid around the world is for 2×2 in. (5×5 cm) slides, the projection facilities being widely available. As ideas and technology change, however, other aids may come to the fore.

When giving a lecture try to use additional techniques and demonstrations to maintain interest; an overhead projector for instance can become one of the most fascinating of visual aids, as dynamic activity is more likely to receive attention. Similar effect can be obtained for smaller audiences with a blackboard or a flip chart. Film and video are excellent communication media, but availability and compatibility of projection equipment must be assured before relying on this material. As well as the local facilities and the size of audience, the type of audience must be taken into account. A group of experts is primarily interested in hard numerical data, although this should be presented in the most interesting way possible. At the other extreme, a junior or naive audience is best introduced to a new field by colourful, varied, and dynamic aids, the number used depending on the amount and type of information presented and the time available. Some material lends itself to dynamic visual presentation, such as by video rather than static slides, particularly practical techniques and the demonstration of physical signs. However, the critical question when preparing material for a specific talk or lecture is whether the necessary projection facilities and time are available. The handout for the meeting will indicate any special facilities available or absent, and if in doubt telephone or contact the organizer at an early date. Visual aids should be available in time to use during rehearsal of a talk. In this way they can be seen to be appropriate, and sufficient time will be allowed for their inclusion, also for any modification. All visual aids must be able to be seen clearly from the back of the hall.

Slides

The 24 × 36 mm colour or black and white film from a 35 mm camera, when mounted, form the standard 5 × 5 cm (2 × 2 in.) slide: these are the basic visual aid for the majority of lectures and meetings. Slides are versatile, easily obtained, easily transported, and reasonably robust. They can be readily stored and sorted. Compatible projection facilities for their projection are almost universally available. Slides are relatively cheap to produce and can be quickly developed or reproduced. Facilities are also available for 'instant' slides using a polaroid process or photocopying techniques. However, these should only be used in emergencies, for example 'off the press' results, since they do not compare favourably with standard colour or black and white slides, and are less durable. Glass mounts are preferred to cardboard mounted slides, as they protect and maintain the film in a uniform focus. However, glass slides can easily be damaged and care must be taken not to scratch or break them. Before use, slides should be cleaned and checked to ensure that they are correctly mounted, with no light projecting around the edges of the film. If possible, they should be set up in a personal container appropriate to the style to be used in the meeting, and taken in this form. The Leitz kind of container requires a special box for transport but great care must be taken to prevent any slides falling out when removing them from the box and when handling them over to a projectionist. The carousel container has a locking top which is more secure, a small piece of Sellotape placed across the side ensures that it does not come undone. If these mounts are not available, slides should be transported in a rigid folder or slide box and never dropped. A number of varieties of folder are on the market, when opened the slides can be identified through the plastic. Examine each variety and decide which best suits your needs. Each slide should contain a single message and should need about a minute of the presentation to discuss, thus about six to eight slides will suffice for a 10-minute paper. More may be acceptable under certain circumstances, for example an operative sequence or when a detailed description is only required on the first of a series of slides. If a single concept produces overcrowding on a single slide it is better to divide the material into two or more slides. A diagram of the method used, and the form of the experimental protocol, is a useful way to start a presentation, as many of the audience may be unaware of these. A photograph of an original recording should also be included to show the quality of the record. Results are best illustrated by graphs and summary tables, while a printed list of conclusions can be of value, provided it is prepared along the lines suggested in the following paragraphs.

Unless he or she is a talented artist, a researcher is wise to enlist the help of an art department to prepare diagrams. However, good originals are essential and care and effort must be taken in their preparation. This rule also applies to photographs and radiographs. A line diagram is often more informative than a photograph, particularly if the latter has not been specifically taken to demonstrate the point being made in the talk. When developing a theme, a series of illustrations can be very informative, progressively adding to a diagram, possibly by using additional coloured material. The area to be photographed in a radiograph should be marked with a grease pencil; a rectangle with of a 3:2 ratio is appropriate. An additional X should be placed outside the lower right-hand corner of the marked area to indicate the way up and the way round to mount the photograph. Word slides require particular care in their presentation. Using these as an *aide-mémoire*, and to include and read out as long sentences, produces an unacceptably dull result. Instead, in a few words, they should provide a clear precise message, quickly and easily readable from any part of an auditorium. There is no point in projecting illegible material and it should not distract, but concentrate attention on the spoken word. If well-prepared, the speaker can assume that the audience sees and reads the contents, and allow a moment of silence while this is taking place. The talk should reinforce and expand the contents of the slide or vice versa; reading the contents is only undertaken for statements requiring specific emphasis. The use of word slides, therefore, requires careful matching of the written and spoken word, particularly with lists, such as a series of conclusions. A long list must be spread over two or more slides and a few written words for each item can be expanded by the speaker into a short sentence.

The number of words on a slide should not exceed 20, 13 being ideal; more than seven lines or four columns should be avoided. The final layout should lie within a 12×9 cm area or an A4 sheet. Lines should not contain more than 32 characters (counting letters and spaces) avoid punctuation marks and underlining—use bold or italics to emphasize key words. Lists are better introduced by asterisks, squares, or circles than by numbers—the latter are less attractive and can be mistakenly taken as part of the text. The type should be bold enough so that a slide can be read easily when help up to the light: usually capitals of 3 mm. Lower case is easier and quicker to read than capitals, but capitals should be used to begin the lines and for proper names. A 10 to 12 point sansserif typeface from an electronic typewriter, with a new carbon ribbon, and typed on A4 matt cartridge paper provides satisfactory preliminary material. This can be enhanced by placing a reversed sheet of carbon paper behind the typescript. Composing typewriters, laser printers and Letraset, provide better contrast, but are not so readily available and are more expensive forms of production. Text should be evenly placed around the centre of a slide, the long axis is placed horizontally unless a five to seven line list is required.

Adherence to these simple rules will ensure that the majority of the audience can read a slide when it is projected. Try not to include too many numbers on a slide—there is no place for projecting tables from the speaker's or any other publication. A few selected values from a table may be rewritten into three or four columns and provide a useful slide to indicate results and trends. Avoid using vertical lines: if horizontal lines are needed, the chances are that an additional slide should be produced. Usually, however, results and trends are better managed by graphs and histograms. Restrict the presentation of statistical data to significant findings and again consider whether they would be better presented graphically.

Graphs differ from those of published material in that long headings and captions are omitted, scale markers and numerals can be reduced in number and headings on both axes are printed horizontally, but the zero baseline must never be omitted. Three or less curves should be included on any one slide and the symbols used to plot the points should be simple, such as circles, triangles and squares. Lines are broken for the symbols and when they cross each other. The same symbols should be used in related slides. Curves are most easily seen when their average slope is 45°. Although individual curves may be widely divergent, the scale should be adjusted to obtain optimal visualization. The thickness of all lines and text must be such as to allow for subsequent photographic reduction.

The rapid expansion of the availability and quality of monochrome and coloured computer graphics is providing an alternative to art work: 35-mm reproduction of high quality displays provides a rapid way of reproducing current and updated results. This facility is likely to continue to improve and the researcher must keep abreast of the available software slide making programmes. Make the diagrams and illustrations interesting and varied, colour adds to a presentation and can be useful in differentiating between groups of results. Use clearly distinguished colours, two are ideal, and not more than four. Be consistent with their use on different slides, repeated changes will detract from the text. Black on white slides are easily read, though less widely used, if they are included for all word slides and diagrams, allow the background lighting to be raised during the presentation. Generally match the brightness of slides to other photographic material, black letters on a light coloured background paper is a useful alternative. White on a blue background slides, can be easily read and are well accepted: they fade in time but usually the colour outlasts the value of the slide. If the same slides are to be used with subsequent additions it is better to reproduce all slides as a new series. Coloured letters produced with coloured dyes or gelatine overlays on a black background can be very attractive. Be sure that these are pale colours, since dark reds and dark blues can be difficult to read; lighter combinations of these colours, or yellow and green, are ideal. At all times consider the presentation as a whole, the balance of colours and renewing old slides to match. If using double projection or 'fade in' techniques do not mix vertical and horizontal mountings and be sure that dual facilities will be available. The two projectors move simultaneously and if information is to be repeated or is absent from one series, duplicate, blank or dark coloured slides must be inserted. Double projection can enhance a presentation, but it is not for the novice, and can court disaster for the inexperienced.

Time must be allowed to prepare, project, and check slides well before the date of a presentation, ensuring that there are no inaccuracies, misquotations, or spelling mistakes, as these must be corrected before the meeting. If a slide is to be used twice, a duplicate must be made and placed in the appropriate position in the series. Although the number of slides in a preparation should be limited to essentials, it is perfectly acceptable to prepare back-up slides in anticipation of any questions or discussions. These should be available to illustrate set points and not form the basis of a second paper.

Overhead projectors

Overhead projectors are readily available in university environments as they form a useful and much used technique for small-group teaching, and are preferred by some lecturers to a blackboard. Their use in open meetings and for larger audiences must be more selective. The projector must be suited to the auditorium and regularly serviced. It must be adjusted to fill the screen and be in focus. The usual size of 10×8 in. (25×10 cm) transparencies must be projected onto a large enough screen to be seen by all the audience. The '8H rule', indicating that the maximum viewing distance of members of the audience from the screens should be eight times the height of the projected image, is a useful guide. Powerfully lit overhead projectors are available and can project to audiences of many hundreds, but they may also dazzle the lecturer, who is looking at the transparency, and the audience looking at the screen. Nevertheless, overhead projectors provide a good deal of freedom of presentation. A lecturer may prepare transparencies ahead of time or during the presentation, adding a dynamic element to the talk and increasing attention. Each frame must be thought about in advance and follow similar rules to those laid down for slides. Each should have a single clear message laid out in an uncluttered, easily visible and legible format. Colour is one of the attractions of the technique and must be freely used. Have two to four coloured pens available to emphasize headings, and differentiate areas of diagrams and curves of graphs. Sequential overlays, building up illustrations, is an informative technique and text may be sequentially revealed by gradually withdrawing an opaque overlay.

Letters must be at least four times the size of those advised in preparing slides (40–48 points versus 10–12 points: 1 point equals 1/72 of an inch or 0.35 mm). This means that typewritten scripts are unsuitable and illegible to an audience of greater than 40. Standard typescript also looses edge definition on enlargement, thus a composing typewriter, Letrasetet, or handwritten material must be used. As with slides, computer graphics are becoming an increasingly important means of presenting experimental data for overhead projectors. Care must be taken not to smudge pen-written material, avoid getting it wet as it may run. Although it is possible to photocopy onto a transparency, coloured photocopiers are not freely available and colour is one of the attractions of the technique. Some transparencies can be purchased with interleaving paper and this should also be used for storage and transport. Make sure that the transparencies of a series are placed in order. Decide which side of the projector to stand and where to lay down the set of transparencies, both before and after projection. If illustrations are to be drawn during the presentation check that empty transparencies, or a clean freely running transparent role, is available, that the pens work, and the projector is set up properly. Write a few letters and draw a few lines to check the size and focus before the start of a session. Be sure that text and figures have been practised, thus avoiding spelling mistakes and running out of space to complete words or figures. When talking from an overhead projector, always face the audience and point to the transparency, not the screen.

Black- and whiteboards

Blackboards have been well-tested over a number of centuries and are widely available. When the blackboard can be easily seen by all the audience, the medium provides an excellent opportunity for the skilled illustrator to actively build up diagrams, using light coloured chalks and broad lines. The board must be fully cleaned and, if it becomes shiny or reflecting, be resurfaced. Good quality chalk is needed: dustfree wax chalks unfortunately produce a shiny board in time and become more difficult to use. The duster must be appropriate to the surface. Illustrations should be planned ahead of time, practised on a blackboard, and checked from appropriate distances to ensure that diagrams are large enough and all colours can be seen. Text must be large and only a line at a time written down during a talk, to maintain the interest of the audience. If larger amounts of text are required this should be written out beforehand and where possible, covered with another board until required. Check the legibility of such material from the back of the hall before use. Unfortunately, the size of a blackboard is such as to limit is use to a medium-sized lecture theatre. Although activity on a blackboard can be televised and projected, the expense of such an exercise is unwarranted except for a renowned illustrator. Another disadvantage is that the lecturer is looking towards the board and not at the audience during illustration, this contrasting with the overhead projector where the lecturer faces the audience throughout. The whiteboard has similar advantages and disadvantages to the blackboard and has replaced it in some small lecture theatres. Ensure that the angle of an adjustable board does not reflect light onto the audience. Use appropriate markers, as their marks can be removed easily without staining the board, and make sure the lines drawn are wide enough to be seen and are in contrasting colours.

Flip charts

Flip charts are a useful, rapid, and effective way of addressing a small audience. The material may be prepared beforehand or actively illustrated, each sheet being used to develop a single theme. In this environment they can also be used by any member of a group to demonstrate a point of interest.

Film and video

The use of video recordings and film can do much to enhance lectures, and these media can stand on their own as individual presentations. Their value in short papers, however, is very limited as they are time consuming and the facilities required are not necessarily available. Their use, therefore, should be limited to areas that cannot be satisfactorily presented by still photography, possible examples include practical techniques and surgical sequences. The preparation of such material requires expertise on camera, lighting, and possibly sound. Although more expensive, this in itself serves to ensure that more forethought and effort is taken than in the production of slides or the other media considered so far.

Planning

The organization of the filming should be planned well ahead of time. The plan should be set out on sheets of paper, divided vertically. The proposed visual material is written on the right-hand side and the corresponding text on the left: horizontal lines are placed across the page after each sequence. In this way a plan evolves and blank sections are filled in with appropriate material, after discussion with other members of the team. The subsequent stages of filming each sequence and editing the programme are best under the direction of a single producer. If this is to be the research worker, rather than an outside professional, even more planning is required since many different skills are involved. To avoid unnecessary expense, the whole of the plan should be completed before filming commences, although modifications may take place as the film evolves. Lay down a logical order of filming so that in the one or two days allowed, all the filming required in a particular location is carried out on one occasion, even if it belongs to a number of different sequences. This reduces the amount of setting up of camera and lighting equipment. A realistic schedule must be set out and adhered to.

Production

The producer must be fully acquainted with the script and all planned schedules. If participating groups, such as camera, lighting, and sound engineers, receive the material in advance, they can discuss the content and anticipate the needs. Subsequent changes must also be clearly indicated to the groups, so they know what is happening and can work to set cues. Once filming starts the producer must provide precise instructions on the order of events and what is required in each sequence. This includes the activity to be filmed and the positioning of one or more cameras, with the appropriate lighting and sound recording.

Setting up a sequence often takes more time than the filming and the producer has to obtain the desired effect in the time available. This is dependent on knowing what is wanted and tactfully directing all participants, getting them to work as a team. The producer monitors what is coming out of each camera, and thus what the viewer will see, by looking through the view-finder of a cine camera or at a TV monitor. If there is only one camera, alternate views are obtained by repeating the sequence with a camera in a different position. In this case, care must be taken to reproduce identical visual and verbal images for subsequent editing.

In silent films a 3-s cue is enough warning to start filming, but for sound, 8 s (time for about 16 words) is needed. Keep the film running beyond the end of a sequence for a few seconds to allow for continuity of sound, thus facilitating editing. It is better to err on the generous side at this stage. TV sequences are played back before proceeding to the next set. Consider additional long shots or close ups of a sequence that could add to the interest of the final presentation. When there is only once chance of filming the sequence, such as an operative procedure, preparation involving camera position, lighting, and sound, must be tested and approved in advance.

Composition

The activity being filmed must fill the screen, be centrally placed and not have any surrounding distracting points of interest or unnecessary material. The distance of the shot is dependent on the size of the point of interest, but a long shot at the commencement of a sequence, or soon after, helps the audience to orientate. This is also so when introducing a new character or reintroduction after a break. Concentration on the geometrical centre of the screen can become uninteresting. Variety is obtained by placing the point of interest off centre, to one of the four points of intersection obtained by dividing the screen horizontally and vertically into thirds. Do not let the top of the head or the chin of a subject continually be touching the top or bottom of the screen and avoid cutting off the top of a subject's head or the side of their face, except in close up. A good rule is to keep the eyes of subjects two-thirds up the screen, regardless of the distance of the shot. Direct eye contact with the camera, however, is only used when a presenter is talking to the intended audience. If a subject is looking to one side, they should be placed towards the other and if walking or running towards one side, the direction of this movement should be retained if included in the next sequence. When more than one subject or object are being filmed, avoid overlap, such as looking over someone's shoulder at half the head of the second individual.

Illustrations

This material should match the horizontal 4:3 ratio of a film or television screen, 30×25 cm card provides a useful size for filming. The medium used depends on time and money: skilled artists must be allowed adequate time to prepare clear lined, precisely lettered lists, graphs, charts, and diagrams. Faster results can be obtained with the use of poster inks, crayons, and lettering pens. However, poor quality artwork is highlighted on screen and these media must still be applied by experts. Crayoned material is best sprayed and fixed to prevent inadvertent smudging.

Avoid excess and irrelevant material on a card, the lettering and lines must be bold enough for easy viewing and separated enough to avoid them running into each other. This is obtained with a lettering 2–5 cm high (depending on whether small letters, capitals or headings) and four to six lines are included, each with about 25 characters. Photographs should be of a matt finish to avoid reflections. Specific attention must be given to contrast: in black and white films, black or white card is used, with the reciprocal lettering or diagrams. With colour, a pale background with bright coloured illustrations are required. Similar attention to contrast and size is essential when preparing overlying captions for an edited sequence. One of the great advantages of television as a communication medium is the ability to provide movement. This can be achieved by uncovering additional information or adding it by hand with coloured crayons or wide felt tipped marker pens. Simple movable overlays can add animation to a diagram but extended animated sequences require specific artistic skills. All activities must be unhurried, positive, and well-rehearsed. Ensure good even front lighting and shoot plenty of film since illustrated material is often talked over and repeated during the course of a presentation.

Camera

A cameraman is in control of many of the factors considered under composition. The camera is best placed at eye level, horizontal, and at a fixed focus, unless specific effects are being looked for, such as zooming onto a small component from a larger area of interest. It may be necessary to track an activity, but all movement must be as steady and as slow as feasible, to obtain optimal effect.

Lighting

Lighting equipment and techniques depend on whether filming in a studio or on location. In the latter, supplementary equipment may have to be introduced to the existing illumination. The main lighting on a set is usually directed at the subjects or objects from an angle of 30° above the horizontal and 30° to one side of the central vertical plane. Shadowing is reduced by a less intense filler light from an equivalent place on the other side of the vertical, and a back light highlights the outline, making it stand out in the frame. Background lighting is directed upwards and adds depth of field. The colour and intensity of the light sources is modified by positioning, focusing, dimming, shuttering, and adding filters, to achieve the desired balance and effect.

Sound

Sound should match, and never be in conflict with, the picture on the screen. Usually sound and vision appear together but the picture should never arrive first. The volume must relate to the distance and the direction depicted. Microphones must be appropriately placed and out of shot: this may require radio or directional microphones. The sound is adjusted by an engineer who is listening with head-phones, and is also on the look-out for extraneous noises, such as distant telephones or passing aircraft, which may not be noted by other members of the team.

Presenter

The researcher may be the best person to present the programme, as whoever does so must be fully coversant with the material. Professional presenters have the advantage of training in the skills of delivery and will probably become involved in editing the script. They will, however, require coaching in unusual pronunciations and the meaning of some statements. In contrast, the researcher may need to acquire some communication skills. A presenter in direct shot is one of the few occasions when direct eye contact with the viewer is desirable. To hold the audience the presenter cannot glance away, this means learning the script, probably in sections with occasional positive reference to cue cards on a front table. Alternatively, cue cards or a rolling autocue can be placed near the camera: the presenter still appearing to be looking at the lens. However, words must be large enough to match the presenter's visual acuity without apparent straining, and the rate of scroll must match the rate of delivery. A certain amount of rephrasing and ad libbing does occur but key phrases must be remembered and given in sequence, as they may also be camera cues. Presentation requires training and experience to produce a well-ennunciated, relaxed, and reliable delivery, with appropriate inflection and pacing to hold an unseen audience. If the presenter is not in shot it is often better to record large sections in a studio at a later date. In this situation sound levels can be easily adjusted and the recording made over pre-recorded appropriate background noise. The presenter can read from a fully marked script in a well-lit cubicle and the recording can be played back and repeated with less pressure on time than when filming. In live TV the presenter addresses the active camera which has the red light on top.

Editing

In live television the producer is controlling which camera is active and is usually in communication by earpiece receivers with camera, lighting, sound engineers, and the presenter. In this way events of interest can be monitored and a balanced programme presented. A programme may be recorded in this fashion for later presentation. However, in these circumstances, and when the material has been collected from more diverse sources, the possibility of editing is available. The first stage of editing is to look at, listen to, and document all the recorded material. Ideally this is done on a copy with a superimposed time marking, otherwise, great care must be taken of the original material and a stop-watch is needed in the documentation. The material is also matched to the sound recording. Editing is based on the original script. During filming the producer will have decided how to cover each sequence and is now able to see if this material matches its aims. Having seen that it does so, a rough cut and splice is undertaken to bring those pieces of film to be used into the required order. Cuts within a sequence must be undertaken for a reason, perhaps to add variety or break up a long piece of dialogue by showing another view, a different part of the scene, a close up or a long shot.

It is not necessary to stick rigidly with the speaker, insert views of listeners, or surroundings. If these alternate views were considered at the time of filming, the material will be available. Similarly, if more than one camera has been used, a great deal of useful, general views will be on film. It is essential, however, that different views of a sequence must match and this can be difficult if one is looking for filler material from elsewhere. Cuts are generally undertaken on a subject movement, such as standing, sitting or turning, but not during a camera movement, such as a zoom. Double image techniques are very rewarding when the two pictures are related, such as a subject watching a playback of their own activity. The very fact that such techniques are available, however, is not in itself an indication for their inclusion. When moving on in time, perhaps during an operation, one sequence can be dissolved into another, this mix should take 2–3 s. Fading out and in takes longer, but also implies a longer span of time. When dialogue is present it dictates the length of a sequence and it may be impossible to shorten it. In silent sequences, the editor has to decide its length, this may be related to an action or perhaps to writing on the screen. The time required for the latter is determined by reading it out loud at a normal pace and allowing double this time for short sequences and one and a half times for a full screen or a rolling text.

The use of music to fill in silence is a standard television technique but, in scientific presentations, it is generally limited to the beginning or the end of a programme. The greatest difficulty is matching the style of the music to the situation without the listener being aware of its presence. The volume must always be appropriate and when using music at the end of a sequence it should be timed to the end of a cadence.

The foregoing paragraphs relate to both cine film and television, but as the cost of television equipment falls and the ease of editing improves, this facility is becoming much more widely available. Well-edited material can therefore, be considered for use, even in short presentation. Ensure, however that TV monitors are available at the proposed meeting and that they are compatible with the format of the video cassette produced. Be aware of the different systems used in different countries and new developments, such as the high definition video systems currently entering the market. All film and video sequences must be matched to the talk and tried out on a home audience before outside presentation.

Multimedia presentations

The combination of photographic and computer-generated images deserve exploration for those excited by multimedia presentations. The combination of a background picture of a piece of apparatus, a product, or a building, with an overlay of one or more pieces of text or diagrams, depicted in full colour, can be very rewarding, as evidenced by the best of national television presentations. Additional facilities include a divided screen, a built-in cursor, text highlighting, and step-by-step image building. Requirements have to be matched to available funding and, when this is not limited, one should decide whether such a presentation would be better provided by a commercial company with the necessary expertise. Key-pad voting systems allow considerable audience involvement and generate interest and enthusiasm. However, these expensive facilities are wasted unless the presentator has planned the session carefully, and defined questions and areas of debate where the audience can be meaningfully involved.

Summary

1. Illustrated material must equate in quality to the spoken or written word that it accompanies. It may take longer to prepare and must be started early in order to match the scheduled date of presentation.

2. Illustrations in written presentations should generally be limited to those areas where they provide a unique addition to the text. A thesis is an exception, and illustrations should be included of all apparatus and techniques.

3. Illustrations should be double their eventual size with appropriate line thickness for reduction. Symbols should be consistent in related illustrations.

4. Photographs for journals should be black and white gloss and unmounted. Written permission should be obtained for the use of human photographs and, unless unavoidable, these should not be identifiable. Scales must be included on photomicrographs and calibrations of all original records.

5. Illustrations should be numbered consecutively and marked on their back with a soft pencil or with a stick-on label, indicating the top, the author's name, the title and the figure number.

6. Tables provide a concise way of presenting numerical information in written presentations.

7. A slide should contain a single message and written material should not exceed 20 words, 7 lines, or 4 columns.

8. Overhead projectors and black- and whiteboards provide an active and interesting aid to presentations in small lecture theatres. Diagrams and text should be well-rehearsed and the size of material should be easily read from the back of the theatre. Extended text should be written out in advance.

9. Flip charts provide a rapid and effective way of addressing a small audience.

10. The preparation of cine and television material requires extensive planning. A working script with full text and details of all proposed visual material must be completed before commencing any filming. Consideration must be given to camera, lighting, sound, presentation, and the subsequent editing.

20. Grant applications

Overview

Communicating scientific data is now as much a part of scientific endeavour as performing the experiments themselves: it is thus not unreasonable for a granting body to assume that deficiencies in an application will be reflected in the author's approach to the scientific problems. Applications must therefore be prepared to a standard that represents the applicant's full potential. If a form is supplied, one is well-advised to follow the required format, completing all sections within the space provided. To achieve these requirements, type the first draft on a photocopy of the form and proof-read this, and the final copy, very carefully. Ensure that the completed form and all additional documents, such as statements from the department and ethical letters, reach the appropriate offices at the correct address well before any set deadline. It is the duty of all large departments to educate their postgraduate students in the art of preparing grant applications for, as new lines of research develop, the need for further financial resources arises. A number of possible public and private sources exist for such an income, but the information supplied to the granting body must reassure them that their money will not be wasted.

Grant-giving bodies vary considerably in their profile, for example from government funded to local support groups. Government-funding bodies, such as the Medical Research Council in the UK and the National Institute of Health in the USA, are tightly controlled, preference being given to workers from high profile research institutions and students with a big name sponsor are more likely to succeed. Many funding bodies are disease orientated, such as cancer, leukemia, diabetes, and cardiovascular research, while other specialist groups, such as medical societies and journals, limit their support to their own field. Wider spread of topics may be accepted by charities, industry, local hospitals and leagues of friends. Pharmaceutical grants may be specifically linked to the assessment of their own products and care and experience is required to establish the degree of independence that will be given to researchers in such instances. Although lists of charitable bodies may exist, choosing the most appropriate, thus avoiding much wasted time and effort, is usually based on advice from heads of department, supervisors and co-workers.

It is the function of granting bodies to distribute their finances to appropriate candidates. They usually have set rules on the level of funding, the length of support, and the type of individual or team that are acceptable. Examples are support for travelling fellowships, training scholarships to gain specific expertise, links between science and industry or between clinical and basic science, and international partnerships, such as those encouraged by the EC, linking scientists from two or more member states.

Styles of application

The style of a grant application need not differ from other scientific writings; it should be clear, logical, and direct in the approach using minimal jargon. The report should be readable and understandable even to a nonspecialist and the layout appropriate to the requirements of the granting body; remember that the accuracy of the content and the references is essential. The prospective requirements of a grant application, however, do differ from the retrospective reporting of completed experiments. In assessing an article for publication, an editor is mainly considering the data and the interpretation of the material. On the other hand the grant-assessing body will be interested in the choice of topic, knowledge of the field, the proposed methodology, the logic of the sequential approach, and the financial responsibility that the project involves.

Choice of topic

The topic must be related to the research worker's interests and in line with personal and departmental expertise. A complimentary interest of the granting body can be mutually beneficial: know as much about the assessors as possible before submitting an application. Originality is one of the most important features which the granting body is looking for, since one of its responsibilities is to ensure progress in any field. Simple repetition of previous work is not enough, unless evidence is available to suggest inadequacies of earlier material. On the other hand aiming to develop an entirely new field is fraught with difficulties possibly better known to a granting body than to the applicant. Consequently, unless some satisfactory prediction of the feasibility of an application in such a field is given, it is unlikely to be supported. Until the reputation of an applicant commands unlimited support, the choice of topic should, therefore, be directed at a new aspect of an existing field. The topic will often be related to one of the problems encountered in previous experiments, or to unanswered questions or controversial reports in the literature.

Knowledge of the field

Incorporate into the application enough evidence to show a full understanding and knowledge of all previous work in the field, including a concise historical review of the findings which led to the proposed research project. The choice of the literature quoted and the accuracy of the references, both in the text and the bibliography, will have marked influence on the granting body. Remember that the granting body will include experts in the field and possibly some of the individuals quoted. Quote any unpublished work which led to the proposed experiments, be sure to read all the current literature on the topic and be conversant with the work of all individuals currently associated with the same field. If a specific application form is not provided, it is wise to include a curriculum vitae and a list of relevant publications with the application. The granting body is particularly looking for expertise in the field of interest, coupled with scientific and technical excellence. It is important to 'sell' oneself to the assessors and this can be done sensibly without showing any tendency to being overpresumptuous. In this section, above all others, be realistic in the proposals.

Sequential approach

The results of the research cannot be accurately predicated but the likely outcome should be commented on and a logical approach to possible alternative results outlined, avoid aimless ramification. Clearly defined questions must be posed together with the proposed means of obtaining the answers. This organization of selected alternatives will reflect critical insight and understanding of the problem. Include credible and realistic predictions of outcome, with target dates for the completion of each aspect of the study. Outline the methods that will be used, and relate them to pilot studies and the available expertise. Include details of the proposed experimental design, methods of analysis and requirements in terms of staff, experimental animals and apparatus.

Financial responsibility

The amount of money available for distribution by granting bodies will be governed by its resources and policies. It is wise to find out in advance the likely figure a particular granting authority will allow for a project of the type proposed, and what arrangements are made to meet inflation. It is possible that more than one financial source will be needed and this will require negotiation with various authorities. State the resources available in the applicant's own department, or any other with which he or she is collaborating, in terms of space, technical support, and specific facilities. It is important to establish whether the department will be willing to continue to support the project with its attached personnel once a granting body has provided the initial capital. Such a project will have to be in keeping with the academic and political policies of the department, as well as within its moral, ethical, and legal codes.

All granting bodies require a detailed breakdown of the costs of a project, this section will prove to be the most difficult to complete until some experience of costing equipment and salaries has been gained. The personnel, salaries and wages, and accounts departments of large institutes carry extensive expertise in these areas, and applicants should seek their advice in this section of the application. Work out separate capital and running costs and decide over what period the research is to run, this is usually 1–3 years. Full consideration must be given to the need of specific equipment. It is important to discuss the matters of cost fully with the head of the department, particularly as he or she is likely to be partly involved in the outlay, even if only in terms of space, and the research may also involve a team of workers.

Assessment

The assessors appointed by the granting body will be a team of experts, and their responsibility is to protect private or public resources and ensure maximum return for the outlay. They will consider carefully the various aspects of an application as outlined in the foregoing paragraphs. In this way, they will be able to assess previous training, knowledge, and achievements and also the judgement, originality, and ability of the applicants. Particular attention will be given to the design and organization of the proposal. In the design, the choice of subjects, and the form of data collection and analysis are critical. Organizational factors include an awareness of the requirement of budgeting time and money. Safety and ethical considerations must be fully discussed, and all techniques fully justified.

It may be the policy of the granting body to hold interviews, during which a rigorous appraisal of the individual or team can be made, particularly with respect to motivation, knowledge, and understanding. Applicants for a technical fellowship, for example, will be assessed for their knowledge of the underlying technology and the potential of their proposed study. They will not be expected to already posess the technical expertise, in fact, demonstration of the existence of these skills could mitigate against the award. By the end of this assessment, the assessors will be fully aware of the feasibility of the proposed study, the validity of the sequential arguments, and the probability of obtaining meaningful results. Grant applications are therefore, some of the most carefully examined of all scientific writings, particularly when a number of scientists are competing for limited funds. In no other field, however, is the scientist rewarded with such tangible returns. Successful candidates may be required to furnish the granting body with the details of progress. A number of granting authorities require annual reports and regularly review the progress of the projects they are supporting. Any proposed changes in the successful proposal should be fully discussed with the granting body. The support from the granting body should be acknowledged in all publications and they should receive copies of these articles. Regular communications of this type will be noted and may encourage further support at a future date.

Summary

1. The choice of topic is best directed at new aspects of an existing field.

2. The applicant must demonstrate a thorough knowledge of the proposed field.

3. Questions must be clearly defined and a realistic sequential approach planned, together with its methodology, including details of data collection and analysis.

4. Costing must be broken down into capital and running expenses over the proposed period of the grant, and due allowance should be made and specified for inflation. Any additional sources of funding which have been sought or offered must be stated. There must also be an indication as to whether the department will continue to support the project once short term monies have been used up.

5. Assessment of the project is based on: its originality; the scientific interest and potential value; the practicability and suitability of the design, methodology and proposed analysis; and the feasibility of completing the project with the time, money and skills available.

6. A grant application is an integral part of current research and should be included in all research training as it is one of the most testing yet rewarding forms of scientific writing.

21. Refereeing and reviewing written material

Overview

Seniority and experience bring with them additional tasks and responsibilities. These include reviewing written material, usually in the form of articles for specialist journals, but occasionally material from a proposed book submitted to a publisher. An understanding of the processes involved is also of value to the trainee, since it can influence the style and content of their own presentations. Reviewing can be time consuming and require detailed attention. The opinions given must be constructive to both the editor and the author, yet they do not usually carry much in the way of reward, be this in terms of recognition or finance. Nevertheless, this is an important service which should be undertaken by experts if the standards in their specialty are to be maintained.

Refereeing an article

A journal referee carries a privileged position and must assume an impartial role, treating all manuscripts in absolute confidence and never quoting or utilizing the material until it is published. The quality of the articles in any journal is influenced by the skill of its peer review system, usually two referees are used for each article. A referee will have written many articles and be aware of the problems referred to in previous sections. From this knowledge he or she should decide whether an article should be accepted, modified or rejected by the journal. The journal may provide an evaluation form or, commonly, a guidance sheet. The decision is based on a number of factors, they are also considered on p. 168 and are based on an understanding of the various statistical factors discussed in Section B.

The material should be original and important. Experimental design and methods of analysis should be appropriate and the experimental technique adequate to examine the problem under study. The results should be complete, credible, and relevant to the posed problem. Conclusions drawn must be justified by the data and a distinction made between these and any reasoned speculation. Scientific credibility is of the utmost importance. The discussion of the article must be relevant to the problem and any conclusions must be fully substantiated. The paper as a whole must be comprehensible and appropriate to the chosen journal. The referee should comment on duplicated or unnecessary text, on the literary style and organization of the article, and the quality of tables and illustrations. References should be appropriate and without any obvious ommisions. Do not carry out any corrections on the manuscript: if the editor chooses to accept the article, appropriate changes to language and style will be made in-house. Any departure from accepted ethical standards in animal or human studies requires specific mention. Criticism of these various factors must be clearly stated and justified. The editor, and probably the author, will read these comments and both will want to know the essential as well as the desirable changes. Comments intended only for the editor should be typed on a separate sheet. The referee should not contact the author directly as most journals prefer to keep their referees anonymous, and the final decision concerning acceptance or rejection of the article remains with the editor. Anyone taking on such an appointment must be prepared to assess any manuscript within 2 weeks and if this is not possible, or the material is inappropriate to their experience, the material should be returned immediately to the editor with a letter of explanation.

Book review

The review is usually commissioned by a journal and of a published work. Anyone reading the review should receive enough information to decide whether to read the book for themselves. Reviewing prospective book material is considered at the end of this section. Editors allow more time for reviewing a book than an article, but the commission should not be accepted unless the book can be read and the review completed within 4–6 weeks. It is the editor's responsibility to choose a reviewer with appropriate experience and he or she may comment on the reason for the choice in the initial request. A reviewer should not proceed unless they feel that they can give an informed and balanced opinion. Although it is unrealistic to expect a reviewer to read every word of a very large text, enough must be read of each section to assess the written knowledge, and the depth and the quality of the content and presentation.

Start by reading the preface, and any additional information on the dust-cover or the publishers handout. This information should indicate the aim of the work and the intended audience. These factors should be kept in mind while reading the book and in the preparation of the review. When reading each chapter make notes that can later be organized and included where appropriate into the review itself. When starting to write the review check on the house style of the journal so that titular details can be laid out in the required fashion. Begin with one or two sentences on the field of study, followed by the stated aim of the work. There follows a description of the text, the illustrations, and other sections such as the bibliography and the index. At this stage give an opinion on the quality of content and literary expertise.

Next the whole work should be put into perspective in relation to the existing knowledge and literature, together with its relevance, the appropriateness of its aims and the success of the author in achieving these objectives. Look for areas of deliberate or inadvertent omission, and consider the choice of material. Opinions must always be directed at the content rather than the author. Finally, comment is made on the value of the work to the intended audience, whether undergraduate or postgraduate, and whether it should be bought and/or read by anyone else.

It is a sobering thought that vitriolic abuse is likely to increase sales of the work and that many successful books can look back on initial miserable support from reviewers. A book review, however, is one of the more rewarding aspects of scientific writing in that the book can generally be retained by the reviewer. Similar honest and carefully considered opinions must be given when reviewing material submitted for publication as a book. Publishers may request an opinion on the basis of one or two chapters, but, if not provided, the aims of the book and the intended audience must be obtained. Decisions are made along the same lines already outlined. They are best given in writing, although a reviewer may work regularly for the publisher and discussion of the text may be all that is required. Publishers generally give a fee for such a commissioned opinion. The single fact that the reviewer thinks he or she could have written a much better book on the topic should not be a prime factor for advising rejection.

Summary

1. Refereeing articles for journals must be carried out within 2 weeks.

2. Assessment is based on originality, importance, scientific credibility, reliability, and honesty.

3. The editor should receive constructive comments on how the article could be improved or why it should be rejected.

4. Book reviews should state the aim of the work and how well this is achieved. Indicate the intended audience and whether it should be bought and/or read by this or any other group of readers. Opinions must be directed at content and never at the author.

22. Applications, references, and interviews

Overview

Taking up a series of appointments at a junior level enables researchers to work for experts in a variety of fields. These jobs are often of short duration and are looked on as training positions. Promotion to more senior positions is accompanied by longer tenure, wider freedom of activity and, eventually, departmental directorships. The route may include appointments overseas, working with world experts in the field, and gaining exposure to different environments. On a more basic level, the reasons for changing jobs are often grouped under the acronym CLAMPS—challenge, location, advancement, money, prestige, and security. It is wise to sort out the particular features influencing you personally and be prepared to discuss them at an interview.

A few individuals will be 'head hunted' for positions, because of the quality of their research activities, as evidenced by their writings, presentations to learned societies, and invited lectures. Most, however, have to search widely and thoroughly to identify appropriate positions. Use the grapevine of associates, contacted by telephone and at meetings, to identify suitable positions and departments. Telephone calls to the latter determine when vacancies are likely to occur, and journals and other media must be monitored for the advertisements. Invitations to lecture in these departments must be sought and accepted, and provide a chance to see their activities. Departments may accept a research worker who has acquired financial support, but this support is more commonly linked with an institution after, rather than before, selection. Obtaining these positions requires planning and industry equivalent to the other disciplines referred to in this text. Well-documented applications, good references, and sound opinions delivered at interview are required to ensure appointment to a desired position.

Appointment applications—curriculum vitae (CV)

Application forms are often provided for junior positions but more freedom is allowed for senior appointments. The format, however, follows a standard pattern and commences with the full name, address, telephone and fax number(s), date of birth, nationality, and marital status. There follow the headings: training, qualifications, and awards. Training and associated qualifications may start at school or university as is appropriate and these, and the awards, are placed chronoligically. Qualifications include the subject and class of degree and any dates of provisional or full-registration with a professional body. For the headings of 'current and past positions held', work backwards in time, and include the starting and completion dates of each position. It is usual to separate professional appointments from other current or previously held positions, such as president, chair, secretary or treasurer of various boards, committees, or societies. A gap in the professional career will probably be picked up at an interview and the candidate has to decide whether to put in the alternative activity or be well equipped to answer the question when it arises. The next group of headings are directed at a candidate's achievements. They may be requested under the heading of 'other information and remarks'. Each title should contain the word *experience*: common sections are professional, managerial, educational, and research. The order and emphasis of these sections depends on the requirements of the proposed position. It is wise to obtain a job description prior to completion of this part of the application, since the impact of this section provides an important factor in selection for an interview. The section is tailored to the job. The contents of each section should indicate the experience and expertise obtained and the achievements and contributions in each discipline, rather than just listing the positions held. The whole must indicate a well-rounded and trained individual, with initiative and the ability to complete and succeed. Extracurricular activities of note are worth an additional section. Publications should be divided into papers, books, and proceedings and placed chronologically, including a full reference (p. 189). A separate section should be given for works in press, submitted for publication, or in preparation. Excessive numbers under the last two categories compared with published works are unlikely to impress an interview panel. A list of presentations to learned societies and invited lectures may duplicate the published proceedings. List two or three *referees*, as requested, on a separate sheet at the back of the application. Make sure that their titles, degrees, addresses, and telephone numbers are accurate. Each referee must have agreed that their name can be used for a specific job or for a specific period, and they should receive a copy of the completed application and the job description at the time of submitting the application. Be sure to keep a referee informed of progress, success or failure, of any interview. Applications for more senior positions require an additional section on *how the applicant proposes to carry out the appointment*. The candidate draws on previous experience of writing theses, papers, and grant applications to match this challenge. Extensive inquiries must be undertaken as to the needs of the position, its current and previous limitations, and how future developments could be carried out, using the position to its full potential.

While proposing innovation and demonstrating initiatives in professional, managerial, research, or educational fields, a candidate must be realistic in relation to the resources available. In particular, a detailed account of the necessary funding must be included with regards to staffing, expenses, and apparatus and some indication of where this funding will come from. Plans should include the 2 and 5 year objectives and the direction that will be taken in each discipline. The text should be concise and these objectives must match the candidate's ability and previous achievements. This two to five page proposal is placed at the beginning of the application and will provide the basis for most of any subsequent interview. All applications should be prepared on a wordprocessor so that they can be accurately proofed and a final perfect printout obtained. The format should be easy to read with judicious underlining. Allow plenty of margins and print in double spacing. If the printout has to be on a set application form, the spacing should initially be tested on photocopies. Alternatively, provided the application form does not stress the contrary, attach a curriculum vitae to the application form, filling in only the initial personal details on the latter. Printing must be of the highest quality available. A laser printer provides an excellent finish and a variety of size and weight of print for different headings. This will avoid the need for using commercial printers, nevertheless, anything but a perfect result is false economy. Make sure the necessary number of applications are provided and only photocopy if the copier is able to produce high quality material. Binding also depends on what is available: a front and back card are desirable. On the frontpiece, place your full name and the position being applied for, together with the month and the year, in a well-designed format. Preparing an application takes at least 2–3 days and if all the information is not available it can take 2 weeks. The decision to apply for a position must therefore be made soon after it is advertised, to ensure that the application arrives well before the closing date. It is worth keeping the information on a wordprocessor, updating it at regular intervals. Be sure to read through the whole of your curriculum vitae before each job application, since changes have usually taken place and inappropriate statements may exist in many parts of the presentation. Up-to-date copies, perhaps printed on less sophisticated equipment, can be carried around when visiting departments and left with senior members of staff, or the secretaries of those it was not possible to meet. Keep a personal copy, and read through it again prior to an interview.

Referees and references

Providing a reference is an important and usually a privileged task of a supervisor or a senior member of staff. It must be taken very seriously as it may profoundly influence the future of a candidate. In turn, the candidate should choose referees with whom there is mutual respect and never use anyone without first seeking their approval. References require careful composition with precise choice of words and it is essential to support good candidates to the full. These reports, however, must be truthful, as they also influence the reputation of the referee. A balanced opinion is needed by the selection committee, superlatives should therefore, be retained for the exceptional candidate. Derogatory remarks are rarely appropriate. Unenthusiastic comments will be picked up and used to unfair advantage by a committee member who is supporting another candidate. It is important that the candidate should know the level of support to anticipate from a referee: this can be given in general terms at the time of request. If a reference is requested for a poor candidate, the referee has to decide whether a reference should be given or whether the candidate should be informed that any reference will be less than optimal. One has to remember, however, that the candidate may not have an alternative referee and specific problems may not necessarily be translated into another working situation. References may encompass a very individual style. This does not mean that a few, even if well chosen, words of excellence will necessarily help a candidate to succeed at an appointment committee. It is wise to at least consider commenting on each of the following suggestions and match comments to the likely requirements of the appointment. Read the request form carefully: although it may be worded in general terms it may request specific information, such as the general health of the candidate. The referee should state the length of acquaintance with the candidate and in what capacity. Comment on the candidate's knowledge, ability, professional skills, attitudes, and specific capabilities. The latter may include teaching, administrative and management skills and the position may require leadership and organizational experience. A candidate's personality and relation to staff, colleagues, students, or any other groups with which they have contact, such as patients in a clinical practice, deserve attention. The final statement should be a recommendation, couched in what is considered the most appropriate terms and directed at the suitability of the candidate for the proposed position. A referee may ring up any interested party to reinforce the support for a candidate. This allows very frank discussion of all aspects of the candidate's abilities without misinterpretation of any deficiencies, such as further experience required in specific areas.

Interviewing techniques

A visit to a department and discussions with prospective senior and junior colleagues is essential prior to any interview. The visit may initially be to assess the desirability of applying for a position but in highly competitive situations candidates may be requested not to visit until after shortlisting. Travel expenses to an interview may be available, from within the country or from a port of entry when coming from overseas, but they are not usually offered for a preliminary visit. Before arrival, arrange to see the head of the department and all senior members of staff linked with the appointment. This allows staff members not involved with the interview to assess candidates and pass on an opinion to the interviewers. Some comments have already been made on choice of a research institute (p. 13), similar attention needs to be given to any professional environment. Obtain a copy of any written job description before, or on arrival at a departmental visit; read it carefully, as many questions may arise from its content.

It is essential to see the present incumbent of the post and discuss the job description with him or her, together with any proposed changes. Inquire as to the advantages and disadvantages of the position, the experience gained, why the incumbent is leaving and where they are going. Find out the typical timetable or workload, teaching, clinical, and other professional activities, and the amount of independent time for personal reading and research. Identify the line of authority, and the back-up help available on professional and secretarial levels. This is an appropriate time to obtain information on salaries, allowances, study leave, expenses allowed to attend meetings, and holiday allowance. This information may also be obtained from the departmental secretary or some other designated person.

An invitation to an interview must be acknowledged in writing. Attendance must be in plenty of time to find the designated site and arrive suitably attired. Timing and attire are both very personal matters but show enough insight not to prejudice any chance of selection before it arises. On entering an interview room, the chair will usually invite the candidate to sit down and will introduce the members of the committee, however, do not be too offended if this courtesy is not extended. Appear composed and sit down at an appropriate time and place to suit the occasion. It is the committee's job to find out whether a candidate has the necessary skill to undertake the appointment; whether he or she has the necessary motivation to carry it out; and whether he or she will fit into the intended team; especially the latter, as technical competence should be ascertainable from the application form. A candidate should give some thought as to how these factors relate to his or her application. Questions will usually commence with one of the panel talking through personal and historic details from the application form. Such closed questions about factual matters require short specific replies, often yes or no. They soon give way to open questions in which the applicant is expected to give longer replies. Aim to give informative and full answers, emphasize important issues at the beginning and reinforce them at the end, without losing way or waffling in between. Highlight achievements and abilities that may be of benefit to the position. However, be careful not to emphasize proposed costly activities, unless the funding has already been obtained and they are in keeping with the policy of the institution. Even if it does not seem like it to the candidate, there are a limited number of sensible questions that can be asked. The usual ones are considered below and the candidate should anticipate them and prepare some short (1/2–2 minutes) 'set piece' replies. Some questions may be multiple, note the various aspects and respond to the ones which you feel happiest with. When an ambiguous question arises spare a thought that the questioner might not have thought it out either. Try to read some sense into it: vague questions do not demand a vague reply. When difficult or abstruse questions arise, repeating the question or inquiring politely as to some aspect of its meaning, gives some time to think, but do not try this too often. A few seconds silence can also buy time and at least gives the impression that due consideration is being given to the answer. In some fields provocative questions can be expected. Be careful not to look on these as personal attacks, or to react in a defensive or aggressive way. Give a clear response stating any contrary view and why this is held; the questioner may well be of the same opinion. The panel is in control of the interview in its content and timing of questions, but when given a chance to speak and take over this initiative, look at the questioner, and try to build up some rapport and mutual understanding. More general responses can be used to make eye contact with other members of the panel. Always respond to the person asking the question but remember the chair of the panel and its other members.

Packaged answers

Fluent, intelligent, and authoritative answers do not come naturally to the uniniti-ated: the set pieces already referred to require careful preparation. The subsequent paragraphs briefly consider the questions which are common to all appointments. Write down the precise answers for the questions which can be anticipated in any forthcoming interview.

What are your prime achievements and what are your strengths and weaknesses?

Achievements will have been listed in the application form: the major contributions documented should be taken and expanded. These will include specific knowledge and expertise, and professional and research activities. The last item will include reference to publications and previous experience. Also include management and or-ganizational abilities, problems sorted, and projects completed. Indicate the factors which motivate you, such as challenge, responsibility, and successful achievement. This personal salesmanship is carried out in a factual and balanced way, without overdoing it or underselling oneself. Weaknesses should not be admitted to. Instead, state how previous deficiencies have been identified and put right, and how obtain-ing the appointment would be an important step in gaining further experience.

Why do you want the job?

The reason for applying for a position is usually linked with career needs, and a candidate should have prepared a statement of their 2–5 year plans and their long-term career intentions. If it is not obvious why the candidate has applied, expect the question and prepare the answer, outlining the specific benefits which will be obtained from the appointment. Expect questions on: why you are moving; why you have frequently changed positions; and how long you will stay. A positive approach to all these matters is essential: unemployment should be explained and how the time was filled, such as additional courses were attended, experience gained, and skills strengthened.

Why should you be chosen rather than another candidate?

This is another way of asking about qualifications, experience, and achievements, and what a candidate would bring to a position. Planned, balanced salesmanship is again required, with an indication of what activities would be undertaken and the assets, benefits, and specific expertise which would be contributed. Do not compare yourself with any other candidate, since you probably will not know their capabil-ity, and might well get it wrong. All responses should indicate a candidate's enthu-siasm and motivation to undertake the appointment. For more experienced positions, questions will be asked on previous experience of supervision, whether you have hired or fired anyone and what types of decisions you find difficult.

What are the key factors in development of a field of interest?

Specific questions on the knowledge and understanding of a field may be issued in an 'examination' style. If the application is appropriate to the candidate's training, their knowledge should be sufficient to answer these questions. Examination style preparation can also be undertaken, since specific attention will be given to recent advances in the field. The questions may be directed at the candidate's awareness of current literature. In particular, any recent report from a government or an organizing body pertinent to the field of interest, should be at a candidates fingertips, together with the likely changes in the field and its future direction and development.

Questions on personal qualities, personal relationships, and teamwork require a balanced response, indicating the skills in these areas and how any previous inadequacies are being sorted out. Pick out a few examples of team involvement which could be used in such an answer. Decide if examples of leadership of successful projects are worth mentioning. Consider extracurricular activities and the level of attainment, and whether these are worthy of mention. At the end of an interview it is customary for a chair to ask a candidate if they have any questions. There may be specific questions which have come to light during the visit, or during the interview, which could influence your acceptance of a position; these should be asked. It is perfectly acceptable, however, to say that all your immediate questions have been answered during a previous visit and during the interview. Other questions should be very carefully prepared and must not appear challenging or denigrating. Sensible questions include: what are the objectives and requirements in a specific part of the appointment and how they will be monitored. Do not venture into questions on salary or annual leave at this juncture: these can be discussed later if offered the job and if there is room for negotiation. Thank the chair and panel on leaving, and consider preparing a final sentence indicating how the job would fit into your career plan and how you would hope to make a positive contribution if appointed.

If you want the job and it is offered, accept enthusiastically and discuss details of the appointment with any appropriate official who is present. It is at this stage that it is often possible to negotiate salary and conditions. After appointment this becomes much more difficult. This is not the time to be indecisive. One can turn down the offer at this point if there is a specific reason. The committee is then in the position to appoint an alternative candidate. Acceptance, and then turning down a position 1 or 2 days later, is discourteous and will cause offence to the committee members, and may adversely affect future career prospects. If unsuccessful, accept that the committee considers there is a better candidate, whatever the underlying reasons. It is valuable to write down the questions and go over the answers given, if possible with an experienced and understanding acquaintance. It is sometimes possible to obtain feedback from a member of the panel, this can be of great help for future applications. Some jobs are worth applying for even when the chances of success are very limited. Surprising appointments do occur, and the interview experience provides the opportunity to be cross-examined on one's various achievements and be exposed to a number of assessors. This may improve later chances. Attendance is not mandatory after shortlisting, but be sure to inform the organizing secretary as soon as possible if you do not intend to turn up. Failure to arrive when expected is a serious omission and likely to be remembered by all concerned.

Emphasis has been given to the limited number of questions and the standard format of interviews, yet interviewers all too frequently meet candidates who are unaware of the rules. Heads of departments and supervisors should ensure that training is layed on for junior staff, that application forms are checked and modified, and interview techniques are discussed. A mock interview with at least two senior members of staff should be held near the time of an appointment. Questions should be similar to those anticipated and be probing, the answers should be analysed on completion of the session.

Summary

1. Applications should include personal details, current and past positions, and publications.
2. Specific attention is given to prior experience, especially in those disciplines appropriate to the advertised position.
3. A well-researched programme is included in applications for more senior positions, outlining the 2–5 year goals, and the proposed sources of financial support.
4. Referees must receive a copy of the job description and the application. In this way they can target the reference, emphasizing the candidate's specific skills and knowledge which are appropriate to the advertised position.
5. A candidate must visit an institution prior to an interview to ensure that it is appropriate to their needs.
6. The interview panel has to be sure a candidate can do the job, wants to do it, and will fit into the team.
7. The questions asked in interviews can be anticipated and answers prepared in advance. These should be tried out in a mock viva.

Index

writing papers/reports (*cont.*)
    acknowledgements 191
    final copy 195–6
    permission to use material 194–5
    references 191–3
    text 190–1
    title page 189
    typed draft 193–4
  pitfalls 171
  proof reading/correction 197–8

selection of journal 187–8
starting to write 188
see also papers/reports
writing theses *see* thesis
WYSIWYG (what you see is what you get)
    interfaces 156–7

z scores (standard scores) 80, 82